I0781431

Natural Home Remedies

A balanced approach to healing

Rani Bains

Copyright © 1999-2022 by Rani Bains

All rights reserved.

ISBN

Table of Contents

Disclaimer

The information in this book is not intended to replace the advice of medical professionals and does not offer any diagnosis, treatment or claims to cure. Please seek professional advice if you are on any medication or receiving any medical treatment before taking supplements.

This book is not intended to be a substitute for medical advice I recommend you seek independent medical advice before following any of the teachings or suggestions in this book. The author and publisher accept no liability or responsibility in the case of personal injury.

Any supplements and remedies recommended are subject to the manufacturers' recommendations. If you are unsure please contact your medical professional or the manufacturer.

My book of remedies - a balanced approach to healing.
First Edition Rani Bains

I have used natural and complementary remedies for over twenty years to facilitate healing. My son was diagnosed with ankylosing spondylitis from a young age. Ankylosing spondylitis is a rare form of arthritis that mainly affects the spine, hips and legs. This illness just came out of nowhere; his symptoms progressively grew worse until he was unable to walk and he was in unbearable pain. During his stay in the hospital, he was still struggling to walk I was at my wits end. I then read something about cranial sacral treatment for children in a magazine. I was desperate, it was very difficult to see him in this much pain, I arranged an appointment with the therapist and took him out of the hospital and after just one treatment he was able to walk again. I was amazed we continued with the cranial sacral treatment, (TCM), acupuncture and Chinese massage, a change to a more alkaline diet, exercise and other remedies for him to be well again. This really spurred me on in the direction of natural, less invasive methods of healing. I believed and still firmly believe that there is a cure for everything if persistence is maintained in search of a resolution.

Since then we as family have relied mainly on natural healing remedies. Although, I cannot say it was easy we faced a lot of challenges; it took a lot of perseverance and many years to see consistent results as my son was not fully mobile for some time; he suffered side effects of the TNF and painkiller medicines during this time. We did not give up and eventually we saw consistent positive results. I cannot explain the gratitude and happiness I felt when I heard my son running up the stairs; I thought it was my daughter until I saw him! On consultations and confirmation from the doctors, my son has been in full remission from this illness and has been free of all the medicines and painkillers for over five years now. He leads a very active life now as he continues with the exercise, pranayama, yoga and dietary changes.

My mother had always relied upon a lot of natural herbs and remedies that had been passed down to her from her family and I understood the importance of passing these things on.

We found that traditional therapies are used to identify the root cause of an issue; whether the problem needing to be resolved stems from a physical, emotional or spiritual Imbalance. Once the problem is identified, a recommendation is made for a natural remedy/treatment. This traditional approach is especially useful in the case of chronic conditions. As a premise, most traditional practices of healing involve cleansing the system prior to commencing other forms of treatment. Many of the treatments are safely used alongside allopathic medicine to help counterbalance the side effects of these medicines. Most healing systems work on the foundation of balancing the elements of the body as a lot of conditions usually arise as a result of an imbalance in the body. These ancient remedies and therapies generally help to correct the imbalances so the body has a chance to heal itself as a whole. There is an abundance of remedies; some are included in this book. We have tried and tested the majority of the remedies mentioned in this book over many years. Some remedies have been passed on down through the generations. I hope everyone reading this book obtains some value and positive influence from the remedies and complementary therapies mentioned in this book.

Prior to taking herbs and supplements check with your doctor. Your doctor should be able to arrange blood tests for you to check for deficiencies, but more thorough and detailed tests can be carried out by naturopath doctors to check for allergies, deficiencies and digestive issues. I have learned a lot of issues arise from problems in the gut. If advised to take vitamins and supplements ensure they are obtained from natural sources. Please be mindful to ensure that products/therapies are used in moderation – it is important to ensure a balance of everything! This is the case, unless a specific dose has been recommended by a qualified doctor, complementary, ayurvedic, homeopathic or naturopathic practitioner. All products are in a whole form for a purpose. The best way for the body to make use of a product is in its natural whole form. For example, when a particular nutrient i.e., curcumin is extracted from Turmeric, it is likely to cause side effects and is better to consume it in the whole form as turmeric, not as an element that has been extracted and taken separately. Where it is possible consume the herbs whole, rather than in extract form. If possible, use products that are organic, genetic modification free and sustainable. If an adverse reaction is experienced when taking herbs and supplements, please stop taking them as each person is different and individual so the body will react differently in each case. Take regular breaks from herbs and supplements, weekly or monthly. It is essential to unburden the organs and release over exposure; so the body is not over reliant on supplements as the body can produce some nutrients. Also remember the body has the ability to heal itself in the right environment.

When making healthier choices and changes to diet and lifestyle, it can take up to 45+ days to feel positive changes in the body, so patience is required. Some of these remedies may work more efficiently when used with complementary healing technique such as meditation, yoga, pilates, qigong, reiki, tai chi, acupressure, coaching, limiting belief work or another form of energy healing work. Many questions have arisen regarding some of the issues and so are discussed in depth in this book. There is also an area for general remedies.

When choosing a more holistic lifestyle it is important to ensure the right balance for everything to ensure physical, mental, spiritual health and general well-being. Going to extremes will cause a reaction and further imbalances. Fresh air free from pollution and an appreciation of nature and treating the environment well are very beneficial to health. If nature and the environment are healthy then we as a whole have a better chance of living a healthy life.

Drink lots of water, preferably filtered water as this can help with any processing required by the body. Reducing the intake of caffeine supports the detoxification of organs such as the liver, kidneys and the adrenals glands. Many varieties of herbal teas are now readily available and are naturally caffeine free. Eating healthy and intermittent fasting may also be beneficial especially to leave at least 10-12 hours between evening meal and breakfast.

Maintain a positive mind-frame throughout as this supports better and even quicker results. Focus on your good qualities and focus on the same in others. Laughter is the best medicine and a cheerful attitude is beneficial to health in so many ways.

To support the balance of all these elements an honest approach to life is necessary. Positive emotions are essential to change the outlook of life, by showing more appreciation. Gratitude is proven to lift your spirits and bring about a positive attitude. There are numerous benefits in gratitude; so it is worth being appreciative for each and everything in life. A positive state of mind is extremely important in life. Gratitude helps you to recognise that good things exist outside of yourself. Psychology research suggests that gratitude touches on many aspects of our lives; ranging from our emotions, mental, physical health, personality, relationships, social dynamics, career success and health; all of these can contribute to increasing our basic happiness.

Also, try not to judge yourself or others as holding onto blame, guilt, regret, resentment only keep you stuck. It proves useful to try to forgive yourself and others regularly if and when you can. We all make mistakes; are all here to learn; try not to make the same mistakes over again. Wish others well even if they have wronged you if and when you can do so as this helps lift off the heavy burdens that nobody needs to carry. Focus on your positive qualities and try to see the same in others that way you will manifest more of the beneficial qualities. Don't forget to live in the moment and be grateful for what you already have because this can provide a great sense of contentment and help you to increase the ability to feel grounded.

The cells in the body are changing all the time and renewing and regenerating. Over a period of seven-ten years the whole body is able to regenerate itself. It is of vital importance then to eat healthy, exercise, keep a balance and ensure positive thinking. This approach works as a preventative measure against ill health and supports a positive foundation for good health.

I hope this book proves to be beneficial and informative for all its readers.

Anxiety

<u>Ashwagandha</u> – This adaptogen and ancient medicinal herb is of great importance in ayurvedic medicine. Ashwagandha promotes a sense of calm and ease, decreases stress and anxiety. It has been used to treat nervous breakdowns and memory loss.

<u>Bananas</u> contain magnesium and other minerals which provide a relief for anxiety and stress.

<u>Breathing</u> – Good breathing is a major component of good health. Long deep breaths and long exhales are beneficial in receiving enough oxygen into the body and releasing carbon dioxide properly. Correct breathing is useful in anxiety and stress reduction. Breathing through the nose is more beneficial than breathing through the mouth.

<u>Brahmi oil</u> – This special oil is one the most effective ways to reduce anxiety. Brahmi is made from the herbs of Bacopa monnieri and Gotu Kola; it is used as a medicinal herb in the East for thousands of years. It aids relaxation and it is very calming. It can stimulate the thyroid. When used on a long-term basis a person is able to handle stress in a different way as it reduces the fear, fight or flight response to ongoing situations and stress. Gotu Kola should only be used fortnightly and then a break should be taken as an increase in liver toxicity may be experienced with long-term use.

<u>Cranial-sacral Therapy</u> is an alternative treatment, whereby the practitioner uses their hands to gently work on the body; this process assists with the release of stress and trauma as well as in the relief of pain and tension in the body. This treatment can benefit many ailments especially in children, such as ADHD. Gentle compression is applied in the sacrum, bones of the head and throughout the body. Cranial-sacral therapy can support the body's ability to balance, heal and restore itself and is promoted as a cure for a variety of health issues.

<u>Shirodhara</u> is an ancient ayurvedic treatment, when used long-term it induces calming and curative effects. The process involves pouring warm oil, (usually sesame oil or milk and herbs), onto the forehead

for twenty minutes at a time while lying on the back. This process is immensely beneficial for relaxation and to promote healing. People suffering from anxiety find this treatment very beneficial and for those with ADHD, it improves the associated symptoms of ADHD such as hyperactivity. Seek advice from a qualified ayurvedic therapist.

The process of Shirodhara works as the brainwaves respond with the external, gentle, yet repetitive stimulation of the forehead; the continuity of this process slowly eases anxiety. As the warm oil streams onto the center of the forehead, it activates a powerful Ayurvedic energy point known as ajna marma. This same physical point is known in Traditional Chinese Medicine (TCM) as *yin tang* and belongs to a category of acupuncture points termed extraordinary points, or those points which are effective on their own. In both the Ayurvedic and TCM medicine models, activation of this point between the eyebrows is said to relieve anxiety and agitation. No needles are required in this case fortunately! Through this process of shirodhara the powerful energy point in the forehead is stimulated and a feeling of relief and lightness is felt as physical and emotional blockages melt away.

The Shirodhara treatment when used long-term can reduce hyperactivity and stress. As a result of stress reduction, inflammation in the body is reduced; inflammation is a major factor of many illnesses such as arthritis, auto-immune disorders, and other chronic illnesses.

A recent study involving shirodhara treatments concluded that, "The relaxed alert state, after treatment, was co-related with an increase in alpha rhythm in EEG." The alpha rhythm is the brain pattern associated with a decrease in anxiety and an increase in serenity. No wonder the shirodhara treatment has long been prescribed by Ayurvedic doctors for treating generalised and specific anxiety disorders, auto-immune disorders, stress and insomnia.

Reiki – If you are open to the benefits, Reiki can be very beneficial to heal a person from past traumas and various different ailments. Reiki activates energy centre's to open and clear blockages in the different areas of life a person is feeling stuck and may be experiencing obstacles or problems such as health issues, relationship problems and career or finance issues. Reiki may be used as a treatment to relieve anxiety and stress.

<u>Tibetan Rites</u> – This yoga practice induces a sense of calm and reduces stress. These rites when practiced regularly are useful in supporting a consistent positive mindset. Other benefits of this practice include anti-ageing benefits due to the regular exercises of the spines. (Refer to Anti-ageing which includes further benefits of the Tibetan Rites).

<u>Ujjayi pranayama</u> is a breathing exercise and is known to reduce stress and tension and is very calming. Ujjayi breathing may ease anxiety issues and the associated symptoms and acts as an aid to better sleep. Do not attempt Ujjayi if you are experiencing problems with your lungs.

Anti-ageing

Amla – Amla is beneficial for the immune system and provides rejuvenation of the skin, gums and hair. It contains high levels of Vitamin C and other anti-oxidants. It slows down the ageing process, assists in the treatment of throat infections, improves heart health and reduces blood sugar levels. It provides major health benefits when consumed regularly and may be taken as a tea.

Asthaxanthin occurs mainly in seaweed (Haematococcus pluvial); which assists healthy cell regeneration; a reduction in wrinkles and an increase in skin elasticity amongst many other health benefits. This pigment in the seaweed possibly protects the organism from the harsh sunlight, especially the ultraviolet rays from the sun. However it can in some individuals affect the absorption of calcium with long-term use.

Bamboo shoot is rich in many amino acids, vitamins and minerals, especially silica. Silica converts to collagen and nourishes thinning hair, skin and muscles. It supports the reduction of hair loss; strengthens weak brittle nails, bones, muscles and skin. Bamboo shoot supports the vascular system, reduces cholesterol, and prevents heart disease. It supports the nervous system, promotes healthy digestion and beneficial glandular system health.

Blueberries and spinach are good sources of antioxidants and NAD+. The latter diminishes with age and UV exposure. NAD+ is found naturally in the body, prevents cell aging and is responsible for the repair of DNA; and of keeping cells healthy and preventing chronic illness.

Castor Oil may support healthier cell growth in the eyes as well as restore the moisture levels in the eyes. This is due its content of ricinoleic acid, an omega 3, that promotes collagen and skin production. Dry eyes can benefit from key nutrients in castor oil. Castor oil use sustains healthy collagen production and also nourishes the scalp and thinning hair.

Chyawanprash has many health benefits. Chyawanprash acts to sustain the body; is known as a rasayana which means it supplies nourishment to all the tissues in the body; it aims to maintain youth and delay the ageing process as it rejuvenates all seven tissues in the body; including the muscles and skin as well as improve the complexion and promote bone and muscle mass. It can reduce sun damage from UV exposure. Chyawanprash can stimulate the body's immune response to infections as well as act as an aid in purifying the blood to eliminate harmful toxins from the body. Chyawanprash can support healthy functioning of the heart and acts as an aid in normalising blood pressure. It supports the respiratory system with the maintenance of clean and clear respiratory passages; it has the ability to enhance overall strength and stamina. Chyawanprash assists and supports a strong healthy digestive system. It nourishes mucous membranes, nourishes and protects the body's immune system, delays the signs of ageing and protects against free radical damage. Chyawanprash is so versatile and useful, that it also assists to promote healthy blood sugar, reduce cholesterol levels, improve the body's resistance to infections and develop overall strength and vitality.

<u>Diet</u> – A plant based diet rich in fresh fruit and vegetables contributes to the maintenance of a healthy digestive system. It is much more beneficial for health to eat seasonal fruit and vegetables as the seasonal produce supplies many health benefits; provides rejuvenating benefits; as well as provides deep nourishing benefits and valuable nutrients for the body. There are also benefits for the planet. Try and moderate intake of junk food, frozen and fried foods. Try and eat cooked meals within an hour of cooking.

<u>Epsom Salt Baths</u> – These salts are very beneficial for the body, muscular aches and arthritis. These salt baths are beneficial for those with skin issues like eczema or psoriasis. The body is able to absorb the right amount of magnesium from the bath due to the high magnesium content of the salts. Epson bath salts are very good for treating stress; promoting relaxation, rejuvenation and assist digestion, improve nerve function and aid circulation.

<u>Exercise</u> – Regular exercise encourages a sense of well-being; influences hormonal health; improves circulation, assists weight

loss, tones up muscles; and improves posture. Exercise provides a release for stress, tension and harmful toxins. Feel good hormones are released during exercise which make you feel well and happy.

Fresh fruit and vegetables are necessary in the diet to achieve good health. It is essential to consume the maximum amount of fresh fruit and vegetables for cell renewal, collagen, hyaluronic acid production and body, cell and DNA health, repair and regeneration.

Goji Berry – Contain extremely high amounts of vitamins and minerals and anti-oxidants. Goji berries stimulate the pituitary gland and promote the release of the human growth hormone (HGH). Goji berries protect the eyes and rejuvenate healthy skin and youthfulness as well as strengthen muscles and bones. The Chinese have used goji berries for over 6000 years to boost the immune system, protect the eyes and neutralise free radical damage and ageing. Goji Berries contain the highest number of most amino acids found, and are also the only super food to assist in the release of the human growth hormone; as well as supply many nutrients and anti-oxidants all found in a single product. Due to the large amounts of vitamin C present in the berries, taking too much may cause diarrhea in some instances.

Healthy fats – In order to prevent and slow down the ageing process it is necessary to consume the right quantity of healthy fats as it is essential to obtain the right balance of omega 3, 6 and 9. These fats can be found by consuming organic coconut oil, avocado, avocado oil, flaxseed oil, olive oil, sunflower oil, ghee and other organic and natural health giving oils and fats.

Herbal euphrasia (eyebright) is mainly used for medicinal purposes in varying forms such as capsules, essential oil, tea, liquid, tablets, and loose dried leaves. The herb exhibits several activities, including anti-inflammatory, anti-oxidant, anti-microbial, anti-viral, anti-fungal, anti-mucus, anti-epilepsy and antibiotic.

Hydration – It is important to stay hydrated as water is very important to support all bodily functions to ensure a healthy cell turnover. Drink good quality water. Hydration prevents acute and chronic health issues.

Marma Facial – This is an ancient ayurvedic facial/neck, head, shoulder and body massage using specific marma points that act to alleviate and release the buildup of toxins, stress, and stagnant energy. This gentle massage can help nutrients circulate and allow regeneration of face and muscles. Marma Facial involves cleansing the skin, then applying a few drops of oil into the hands, rubbing the hands together to create heat and massage the marma points from the chin, mouth, nose, neck, face and head in an anti clockwise motion, then in a clockwise motion to release toxins and blockages; which are very beneficial as blood and nutrients are encouraged to circulate as this therapy is very nourishing and calming. Maintain the massage until all the oil is absorbed into the skin.

Massage skin – Do this regularly as it can assist the blood flow, aid toxin removal and nourish the skin, it is especially beneficial before taking a shower. Massaging the skin encourages collagen production.

Moringa – Known as the miracle tree, it has many benefits. It aids in collagen production. It contains properties that protect the skin, reduce wrinkles, nourish and stimulate hair growth. Moringa is a diuretic and due to the vitamin C content too much is likely to cause diarrhea and dryness of skin. It may provide relief from sensitive teeth and gums when rubbed into the gums with oil regularly. Moringa has been used for thousands of years in the east as it is very nutritious and rich in healthy antioxidants. It contains anti-inflammatory properties and bioactive plant compounds.

Neem – This ayurvedic herb has many properties some of those include its use as an anti-bacterial as well as an anti-fungal. It possesses anti-oxidant and anti-inflammatory properties that fight oxidative stress which in turn may promote liver and kidney health. It may boost dental and oral health, improve skin conditions as it supports the radiance of skin when drank as a tea first thing in the morning.

Qigong – This practice assists the body to build healthy bone density, slows down the ageing process and improves health. It activates the acupuncture meridians, and assists balance; it can strengthen internal organs; enhance power, reduce stress, promote relaxation as well as aid sleep and healing. Bone density is improved due to this practice so it is extremely beneficial in injury prevention and the qigong practice provides the necessary support for injured parts to heal more quickly.

<u>Sensitive teeth</u> can be re-mineralised by gently massaging teeth and gums with mustard oil and salt. This oil has anti-bacterial and anti-inflammatory properties and used with Himalayan salt at least twice a day is really beneficial. A noticeable difference is felt within a week. Moringa may also be rubbed into the gums due to its beneficial anti-bacterial properties as well as its collagen enhancing properties.

<u>Shatavari</u> – This is a hormonal balancing herb, it is especially used as an aid for women's health. Shatavari can be made into a paste with water or coconut oil and used on wrinkles.

<u>Shea Butter</u> – Due to the natural occurrence of chemical compounds within this tree nut, the butter obtained from it provides a unique balance of oils and vitamins to fully nourish the skin. These naturally occurring chemical compounds are thought to deactivate collagen fibre destruction and minimise the appearance of fine lines and result in more youthful, plumper skin. Shea butter also helps to promote cell regeneration; it's moisturising, and anti-oxidant properties work together to help the skin generate healthy new cells. As the body is constantly regenerating and making new skin cells and getting rid of dead skin cells, and can actually get rid of 30,000 plus old skin cells each day. Dead skin cells sit on the top. New skin cells form at the bottom of the upper layer of skin (epidermis). With the right moisture balance on the surface of your skin, there are fewer dead skin cells in the way of fresh cell regeneration in the epidermis. Shea butter may reduce photo-ageing — this is the damage to skin that environmental stress and ageing can create on skin such as wrinkles and fine lines.

<u>Skin</u> – Massage body and face skin in the morning with almond oil, before taking a shower and keep skin clean and hydrated. Eat lots of

fresh fruit and vegetables every day and drink plenty of good quality water. Ensure consumption of good healthy fats to keep skin and muscles toned and healthy.

<u>Tibetan Rites</u> – This yoga practice has been used for centuries to slow down and even reverse ageing. There are five yoga poses combined with the breathing techniques, each of equal importance and are known as a way to reverse the many physical impacts of ageing. The anti-ageing benefits of the five Tibetan Rites have led to them being referred to as The Ancient Secret of the Fountain of Youth.

<u>Turmeric</u> it is a very powerful spice and may be used in the prevention of ageing. Turmeric used as a facemask with honey offers many benefits to the skin; it supports the cleansing and regeneration functions of the skin. Due to all the vitamins and minerals such as copper, turmeric delays ageing, acts as a support to stimulate the brain and prevents neurodegenerative disorders. Turmeric used in the bath with milk will make skin more youthful and radiant as the <u>Copper</u> contained in the turmeric has numerous benefits such as it stimulates the brain, prevents premature ageing, improves functions of the thyroid gland, assists in the healthy production of blood cells, supports the maintenance of bones, nerves and blood vessels as well as support the production of hair colour pigmentation. Although taking turmeric dry without milk or fat may create heat in the body so use in moderation to avoid excess heat in the body. This herb is a very effective anti-inflammatory and can be used to remedy arthritis and other inflammatory conditions.

Arthritis

The symptoms of arthritis are closely associated with joint pain and stiffness. These symptoms may worsen with age. This condition causes the swelling and tenderness of one or more joints. The most common types of arthritis are osteoarthritis and rheumatoid arthritis.

Osteoarthritis causes cartilage, the hard tissue that covers the ends of the bones where a joint is formed to break down. Osteoarthritis is a quite a common condition which can affect any joint in the body, generally it affects the joints that bear most of our weight, such as the knees and feet and the joints of the hand. It is mainly the joints that are used regularly that are increasingly exposed to this condition.

Rheumatoid arthritis is a disease which in the beginning affects the lining of joints. This is also when the immune system attacks the joints.

Where too much uric acid is present in the blood stream; uric acid crystals form that can cause gout, infections or underlying disease, such as psoriasis or other types of arthritis.

The main intentions of arthritis treatments are to reduce arthritis symptoms and improve quality of life. Treatments vary depending on the type of arthritis. Urgent medical attention is usually recommended in severe cases by healthcare providers and arthritis can last several years or last for life.

Complementary and alternative medicines are available as treatments for arthritis, gout, osteoarthritis, rheumatoid arthritis and other joint pain and inflammation. As these treatments are more natural, people generally feel more in control especially for those with persistent pain, without the concerns about the serious side-effects of medication. As many times the symptoms of arthritis are not fully controlled by modern western medicine. There are many alternative herbs, medicines and supplements as discussed throughout the book. The effectiveness might be judged by measurable improvements in the condition or general well-being but it also may relate to whether you feel improvements from the symptoms and the severity of the condition.

Chiropractors and osteopaths may be able to assist with the relief of some of the symptoms of arthritis. It's difficult to say which complementary and alternative therapies would work for an individual, as everyone responds differently to the treatments. Many of these therapies require active participation and a certain amount of positive belief in the possible outcome. The practice of self-care and stress relief is very essential for managing chronic diseases like arthritis. Numerous healing modalities are mentioned throughout such as cranial sacral, pranayama, shirodhara and other treatments as well as herbs which are useful for the relief of inflammation, pain and stress – yoga, qigong and meditation are especially useful to ease these symptoms.

Some arthritis patients regularly use Epsom salt baths to assist with the relief of arthritis pain, as soaking in Epsom salts can provide considerable pain relief and healing for arthritis sufferers due to the magnesium content and a reduction to the severity of other associated symptoms. Soaking in warm water with, ginger or turmeric and bicarbonate may assist with the reduction of inflammation, pain and stiff joints. Ginger, turmeric and bicarbonate are also acid neutralizers and are all alkaline. These herbs are very powerful, anti-inflammatory agents. Turmeric especially is very powerful and beneficial as it is used to remedy arthritis and many other inflammatory conditions.

Other mineral baths may also prove useful to provide relief pain and relaxation, as the distinctive scent of many mineral baths is from sulfur, but magnesium is also present in most natural springs. Other minerals may also be present, which support the balance of electrolytes in the body. Important electrolytes need to be replaced as the arthritis medications can sometimes cause sickness and diarrhea; as a result important electrolytes are lost. These baths are a good way to replace the lost electrolytes.

People have since ancient times found relaxation or pain relief by immersing themselves in warm mineral baths at natural springs. There are also many physical benefits to bathing in warm water to relieve arthritis, chronic pain and inflammation symptoms. The heat from the water is very soothing to stiff joints. The thermal and mechanical benefits of warm water are well-known and include muscle relaxation, improved joint mobility and reduced pain.

A focus on diet can assist arthritis symptoms; a switch to an alkaline diet and a change of diet to include anti-inflammatory foods may provide some relief.

- A change to anti-inflammatory foods is said to reduce the risk of disease that is associated with chronic inflammation.

- This diet emphasizes including more fruits, vegetables, protein, nuts, seeds, and healthy fats.

- It can potentially help reduce inflammatory markers and assist long term and chronic inflammation.

- Certain foods contribute to inflammation in the body, for example trans fat and refined sugar, along with certain meats, (due to their saturated fat content). Saturated fat can cause certain immune cells to release inflammatory proteins into the bloodstream.

- Certain foods however do not trigger this effect and in some cases, they can actually reduce inflammation. This includes the foods that are rich in anti-oxidants. Anti-oxidants fight chemicals known as free radicals that cause long-term damage to cells and an increase in inflammation.

- Food choices influence the level of inflammation in the body, the anti-inflammatory diet is thought to curb chronic inflammation and assist with the prevention of conditions like arthritis, heart disease, and other diseases. There is some evidence of the benefits of this diet, although it's not known exactly how much the diet can help.

- An anti-inflammatory diet led to a 37% decrease in inflammatory substances, such as C-reactive protein, (CRP), in people with type 2 diabetes after just one year, according to a 2016 study.

There are however foods that should be avoided, as these foods cause an increase in inflammation. These foods include those that are high in omega-6 fatty acids. These fats are essential to bone health, brain function, and metabolism (the conversion of food to energy), consuming too many omega-6 fatty acids can increase inflammation. Foods high in omega-6 fatty acids include: High-fat dairy products (such as, cheese, butter, ice cream and milk); Margarine; Meats and Peanuts.

In order to keep inflammation under control, it is important to balance the omega-6 fatty acids intake with the intake of omega-3 fatty acids.

Omega-3 fatty acids are the good fats; they offer assistance with protection against arthritis, heart disease and other conditions. Foods high in omega-3 fatty acids include: Flaxseed, Omega-3-fortified foods and walnuts.

The food with a high glycemic index (GI) can also increase inflammation. These are the foods like sugar and refined grains that raise the blood glucose (sugar) level too much and too quickly. To assist with the management of inflammation, avoid sugary drinks, white bread, desserts, and processed foods. Instead, eat low-GI foods like, leafy greens, whole grains, and non-starchy vegetables.

Over time studies carried out on arthritis patients have suggested that people who eat lots of vegetables, fruits, nuts, seeds, healthy oils, have a lowered risk for inflammatory-based diseases. The substances found in certain foods, especially the anti-oxidants and omega-3 fatty acids, also have anti-inflammatory effects. The foods high in anti-oxidants include: for example fruits and vegetables such as apples, artichokes, avocados, beans, (such as black beans, pinto beans, red beans), berries (such as blackberries blueberries, raspberries), broccoli, cherries and also dark chocolate (at least 70% cocoa), dark green leafy vegetables (such as collard greens, kale, spinach), nuts (such as almonds, hazelnuts, pecans, walnuts) and sweet potatoes and whole grains.

There is also evidence that certain herbs and spices, such as ginger, lemon and turmeric can alleviate inflammation, as well as the regular use of apple cider vinegar. Many claim apple cider vinegar (ACV) and honey, assist with their arthritis symptoms. Acv is alkaline in nature. Vitamins and minerals are essential nutrients to ensure healthy functioning of the body; enrich the diet with foods that are essential in the reduction of inflammation with nutrients and vitamins.

Vitamin B5 for arthritis – Pantothenic acid is available in a variety of foods. Rich sources of pantothenic acid include, yeast, broccoli and whole grains, milk, yogurt, legumes, mushrooms, avocado and sweet potatoes are also good sources. A number of studies have indicated that this is a useful supplement for the treatment of arthritis. Vitamin D is essential for healthy bones.

Flaxseed oil is a vegan alternative; it contains omegas 3, 6 and 9, together, palmitic acid, stearic acid and is rich in ALA. This fatty acid assists in reducing joint inflammation; evidence shows this as an effective treatment for arthritis.

Other supplements to alleviate the damage to the body from arthritis include:

<u>Glucosamine</u> is naturally found in the human body. Glucosamine occurs mainly in the body's connective tissue, (it is an amino sugar), which is a synthesized form of glucosamine. This vegan compound is used to treat several diseases in the human body, especially arthritis. It plays an important role in the production of certain proteins and lipids in the body. It is very important that joint lubrication is maintained and this compound assists to increase the production of hyaluronic acid which is a component of synovial fluid. This fluid assists in joint lubrication. One of the most important glucosamine benefits is its use in arthritis treatment. It is used to ease the pain and to get rid of the symptoms of arthritis by rebuilding cartilage in the body.

It can be taken in combination with Mythocondro (Chondroitin), and with MSM. MSM is a natural sulfur compound that is essential to carry out different functions in the body. The three are available in the form of dietary supplements and tablets. All three are sometimes used in a combination for greater effectiveness in treating diseases such as arthritis and should be taken with the naturopath or doctor's consultation. Vegan Mythocondro and Phytodroitin – (Chondroitin), especially, helps in slowing down the progression of arthritis. In combination Vegan Glucosamine chondroitin also aids in treating the inflammation caused due to arthritis.

- Glucosamine chondroitin assists to increase the production of hyaluronic acid which is a component of synovial fluid. This fluid helps in lubricating joints.

- One of the other glucosamine sulfate benefits is that it is used in the human body to help build cartilage.

- Glucosamine chondroitin also help in enhancing the repair process of the body naturally.

- When compared to the animal-derived product, the glucosamine chondroitin vegan source offered a significant reduction in positive mediators of inflammation. This may be due to vegetarian or vegan preservatives in the supplements as opposed to artificial preservatives and fillers.

There are no known severe side effects. However, in some cases glucosamine can lead to temporary gastrointestinal disorders, diarrhea, nausea, etc. On the other hand, some glucosamine chondroitin is believed to lower the level of insulin in the body. Therefore, people suffering from diabetes are advised against consumption of this dietary supplement.

- MSM, (Methylsulfonylmethane), is organic sulfur. MSM is found in many fruits, vegetables, grains, and milk; unfortunately the amounts are reduced in these foods during the cooking process. It is available in vegan supplement form. MSM reduces pain, inflammation, and allergic reactions. MSM reduces the severity of auto-immune disorders due to its anti-inflammatory, analgesic, detoxification, mucosal healing, and anti-oxidant effects; MSM helps to reduce auto-immune reactions, particularly in and around joints and connective tissue. It also has wound healing, dermatologic, and exercise performance enhancing effects.

MSM is sometimes combined with other supplements such as Glucosamine Chondroitin. There is evidence that MSM in combination with other supplements may assist with the reduction of the pain and swelling of knee osteoarthritis. Also, early research shows some promise for decreasing joint degeneration. Studies also show that MSM may assist the body to heal after exercise recovery.

Another benefit of MSM includes promotion of healthy joint function by reducing swelling and pain to also aid in improving the flexibility of the joints. MSM can be taken in small doses daily for osteoarthritis. However, optimal doses of MSM have not been set for any condition.

So far, studies have shown minimal side effects when MSM is taken orally in small dosage daily for six months, but some people may with higher doses experience mild gastrointestinal side effects such as discomfort or diarrhea.

There doesn't appear to be an interaction between MSM and medications, herbs, supplements, or foods.

Digestion

<u>Bhringraj</u> has exceptional properties which are useful in case of indigestion issues and constipation.

<u>Constipation</u> – This is alleviated by eating fresh fruit and more raw or steamed vegetables regularly. Eating figs, prunes and taking prune juice will help with regular bowel movements. Drink enough water daily, drink caffeine free fluids such as fennel/peppermint tea frequently throughout the day.

<u>IBS</u> (irritable bowel syndrome) the symptoms of IBS include abdominal pain, cramps, food sensitivities, gas bloating, constipation and diarrhea. Aloe vera is from a succulent plant species of Aloe. This plant is very beneficial for this condition; it is the recommended treatment for IBS as it eases gut inflammation. By eating sensibly and avoiding the foods that trigger this condition inevitably will assist with the prevention of IBS symptoms. Other herbs that may reduce IBS symptoms include chamomile, fennel, lavender and mint. Probiotic foods ease the symptoms of IBS. Triphala taken regularly assists IBS, especially if the main symptoms are constipation; it can assist with the repair of a damaged gut.

<u>Clear toxins</u> – Eating kitchari, (rice and split moong daal), will rid accumulated toxins and congestion from the mind and body tissues. Eating kitchari will remove heaviness and congestion in the body when eaten regularly. Kitchari provides nourishment for the body; aids digestion and assists regular bowel movements. This cleansing food supports a healthy body and weight. When eaten regularly long-term it will improve health conditions and allow assimilation of nutrients.

<u>Other digestive issues</u> may be resolved by eating real food and avoiding processed foods. It is important to ensure there is enough digestive acid, digestive enzymes and that good gut bacteria are healthy, (naturopath doctors offer regular tests to determine the balance of gut health). If digestive acid/enzymes/ healthy gut bacteria are lacking, it may be difficult for the body to digest food properly, the body may be unable to break down food and absorb nutrients fully. The tests will also identify if there is a candida overgrowth and the naturopath will recommend holistic remedies to address this

problem. Drinking CCF tea after each meal aids digestion. Hingvastik a herbal remedy, is usually taken after meals to ease digestion for chronic digestive issues.

Raspberry leaf tea has natural mild laxative properties. Due to its laxative properties it can ease bloating and cramping and make it easier for bowel movements.

Taking Triphala each morning may support the repair of a damaged gut; it is used to heal the stomach and is also taken to get rid of anything unhealthy and toxic in the digestive tract. Triphala is a blend of three ayurvedic herbs, Amalaki, Bibhitaki and Haritaki.

Grey Hair

This is usually due to a reduction in the chemical known as catalase required in maintaining natural hair colour. Over time hydrogen peroxide may increase, resulting in grey hair. Some of the following methods assist with the increase of Catalase:

- Applying Bhringraj oil and massaging the scalp each night and washing out in the morning.

- Big Gokhra plant taken with black sesame seeds, honey and ghee in the morning may help with grey hair reduction. Onion juice massaged into scalp, can be mixed with other oils for absorption to the scalp.

- Coconut oil boiled with curry leaves and then massaged into scalp over time can remedy grey hair.

- Bhringraj and Brahmi both assist in the reduction of hair loss and greying hair. Bhringraj is an especially cooling ayurvedic herb as heat in the crown area can cause hair-loss and premature greying.

- He shou woo – a Chinese herb, taken orally can treat and prevent premature grey hair.

- In the meantime use the water retained from boiled walnut husks as a final rinse after hair wash as a temporary natural hair colour. Bhringraj, Indigo and henna may also be used as temporary natural hair colour. For a more permanent hair colour there are a few more natural hair colouring products available with reduced chemicals.

By addressing grey hair issues in advance you may be able to remedy the problem. Enrich the diet with foods that contain hair vitamins such as: avocados, brewer's yeast, molasses, whole grains, rice, strawberries, kiwi, papaya, melon, green vegetables, potatoes, green peppers, vegetable oils, soybeans, raw seeds, dried beans, wheat germ oil, and most other whole foods.

Grey Hair maybe caused by a deficiency of vitamin b12. For prevention of grey hair the following vitamins may also prove beneficial.

- Vitamin A, this vitamin aids the production of healthy sebum (an oily substance produced by the sebaceous glands that lie beneath the skin.

- Vitamin C, besides all its known benefits, it is an anti-oxidant. Anti-oxidants protect the cells of the human body from oxidation or the damage caused by air.

- Vitamin B-6 and B-12 are two of the Complex-B vitamins that support healthy skin and hair. B-6 may help restore hair back to its original colour following an illness or deficiency.

- Para-Amino benzoic Acid (PABA) and Pantothenic Acid are part of the B-complex vitamins and maybe used to postpone the onset of greying hair. It appears that when Pantothenic Acid and folic acid are taken together this combination helps reverse grey hair by taking the hair back to its original colour.

- Inositol, is a substance found naturally in the human body which may encourage the growth and overall health of hair.

- Biotin produces keratin which is a major component of hair and nails.

- Niacin contributes to scalp circulation which in turn nourishes the hair follicles.

Only take supplements after consultation with a doctor, naturopath, or other health practitioner.

Hair-loss

Several factors contribute to hair loss. Generally, hair-loss may be caused by a deficiency of certain vitamins and minerals, such as iron, biotin, folic acid, copper, zinc, b vitamins, iodine and more recently a selenium deficiency; as soils are now depleted of minerals. Reduce caffeine, as caffeine intake can increase levels of DHT (di hydrotestosterone), in the body. The enzyme 5a-reductase catalyzes the formation of DHT from testosterone in certain tissues and hair follicles. Include nutritional yeast in the diet as this can prove beneficial in the prevention of hair loss especially as it is a rich source of b vitamins and it contains biotin. The use of hormone regulating foods such as maca act to aid the regulation of hormones.

Maca can be combined with avocado oil or olive oil and applied to the scalp prior to washing hair to reduce dihydrotestosterone, (DHT) in the scalp.

For women it may be due to thyroid, menopause or other hormonal imbalances, so it is worth getting these issues checked; generally a reduction in progesterone/estrogen may contribute to hair loss as a decrease in these hormones can lead to hair loss and can contribute to an increase in the production of androgens (shrink hair follicles). An increase in the xeno estrogens in the food chain, can affect hair loss in women, even the use of processed food, plastic water bottles, plastic containers, meats not labelled as hormone free etc can affect hair loss. It is important therefore to increase the levels of progesterone by consuming vitamin B6, iron, magnesium, zinc. Zinc helps the pituitary gland and is beneficial for the follicle stimulating hormone and the reduction of DHT. Progesterone is an inhibitor of the enzyme 5 alpha-reductase; this enzyme converts testosterone to DHT.

The food groups to include in the diet to obtain these nutrients are avocado, carrots, fresh vegetables, leafy greens, legumes, maca, nuts, seeds and yoghurt. Essentially look for ways to reduce stress as progesterone is used in the production of cortisol (stress hormone); therefore high stress levels contribute to reduced levels of progesterone.

- A gentle massage using almond oil, (sesame oil in winter), or coconut oil twice a week can help nourish hair roots, the scalp and epidermis.

- Aloe vera gel applied to the scalp can ease itching and work as a DHT blocker for balding.

- Amla, Bhringraj, Brahmi and pumpkin seed oils are used to reduce hair loss and greying hair. Bhringraj is an especially cooling ayurvedic herb as heat in the crown area may cause hair-loss and premature greying, reduce hair growth and cause baldness: Bhringraj helps to boost blood circulation in the scalp region and hair follicles; this in turn results in more nutrients supplied to the root of the hair.

- As mentioned stress can contribute to hair loss and there are certain relaxation therapies that can reduce stress.

- Haematococcus pluvialis. The red colour is due to the pigment called astaxanthin, which possibly reduces the 5 alpha-reductase enzyme thus reducing the level of DHT in the body.

- Practice Kapalbhati Pranayama as this aids cell renewal. Anulom Vilom practiced for 5 minutes and Bhramri pranayama assist with the prevention of hair loss but must only be learnt from a suitably qualified yoga teacher.

- Certain Yoga asana shoulder and head stand help blood circulation to the scalp. Caution must be given as those with high blood pressure should not attempt some of these yoga asanas and pranayama practices. Tibetan Rites have shown to be extremely effective in reversing hair loss in some.

- The acupressure points for hair are located in the fingernails so by rubbing fingernails together hair growth is encouraged. Do not rub the thumbnails together as hair can sprout from the nose and ears.

To further promote hair growth and reverse hair loss, anagen is the sought-after stage, MSM is thought to either promote the conversion of telogen to anagen or lengthen anagen, mainly due to the deliverance of sulfur to the middle layer of the hair. MSM helps to treat alopecia.

- <u>Apple cider Vinegar</u> has a huge array of benefits and may prevent hair-loss when diluted and applied onto the scalp due to its alkaline nature; prevent hair-loss when diluted and applied onto the scalp due to its alkaline nature; it can balance the ph of the scalp. MSM may reverse hair loss and alopecia.

Avoid chewing or twirling your hair because it will split the ends, leading it to break more easily. Do not spray perfume on your hair because it contains chemicals that will dry the hair out and alter its colour. Increase your protein intake: Plant-based sources rich in protein include mushrooms, pulses, raw unsalted nuts, seeds, spirulina powder, nutritional yeast, and broccoli. Combine pulses with whole grains to receive all the essential amino acids. For better absorption or in case of any digestive discomfort, soak the pulses, nuts and seeds with water overnight.

Hay Fever

<u>Hay fever</u> – This disorder occurs at particular times of the year in reaction to allergens, or sometimes all year round known as allergic rhinitis. Allergens could be pollen, dust, mould and pet hair. The main symptoms include sneezing, watery eyes and runny nose. Homeopathic Remedies include Allium Cepa, Euphrasia and sabadilla.

<u>Allium cepa</u> is most often used because of its ability to reduce the symptoms of hay fever. This homeopathic remedy is derived from red onions. It is used to treat conditions affecting the mucous membranes of the nose, eyes, and throat. It is a popular remedy in the case of allergies such as hay fever and in cases of coughs and colds and it is also used to lessen nasal discharge associated with other allergies and infections. It is also the recommended remedy for either infectious or allergic coryza (catarrhal inflammation of the mucous membranes of the nose). Other symptoms may include sleepiness with difficulty concentrating, or foggy feeling with the coryza. Symptoms are worse in the evening and in warm rooms and are improved by open air. Those needing Allium cepa to a great extent may like onions. This remedy may also be used for: bland tearing of the eyes with burning nasal discharge (where the skin under the nose gets red and irritated). Allium cepa is used when the nose is constantly running and for thin, watery discharge from eyes and nose. Other symptoms for its uses include:

- Hay fever.

- Watery discharge from nose and eyes.

- Acrid, burning, excoriating discharge from nose but bland, watery discharge from eyes.

- Symptoms worse in evening and warm rooms; better for open air.

- Sleepiness and difficult concentration with allergies.

- Colds that move downwards to the larynx or chest.

- Sensation of rawness in nose.

- Pain in larynx on coughing.

- Blisters on heels.

(Note: Inappropriate use of Allium cepa can cause head colds to go to the chest. (If there has been no improvement in symptoms, do not use this remedy beyond the prescribed dosage.)

<u>Euphrasia</u> – Homeopathic euphrasia is one of the more effective remedies available when it comes to treating eye conditions as this remedy is made from the plant known as "eyebright." It is believed that eyebright received its name from a traditional medication for treating eye irritation. The herb eyebright has been used to treat eye strain and inflammation since the middle ages, today, herbalists use it for infections and:

- allergic conditions of the eyes;

- skin conditions;

- sinuses;

- nasal passages and middle ear;

- treat eye problems;

- allergies, measles, and cold symptoms;

- digestive concerns and nausea;

- and sleep problems and memory issues.

This remedy is particularly supportive with the relief of several eye conditions, including blepharitis, cataracts, conjunctivitis, eye allergies, eye strain, granular eyelids, glandular swellings and sties. It is also used for dry, inflamed, and stinging eyes. In these cases, the eyes water profusely with a pungent smell. Coughing, open air, or lying down may lead to intense eye watering, and the tears are hot. Often the eyes are also sticky in the morning. For granular eyelids, euphrasia is helpful when the edges of the eyelids turn red, when there is a burning sensation that makes the eyes very sensitive to the touch.

Other symptoms include enhanced sensitivity to light and a desire to blink consistently. In general, the eyes are red, burning, and bloodshot with itchy eyelids. It may also feel like a hair is irritating the eye. Sunlight and wind make the condition worse and winking and eye rubbing help relieve the eye conditions. Conjunctivitis may form after the flu, measles, injury, or other health problems.

It is also the suggested remedy for eye rashes with unclear vision and swollen eyelids. There is also a pain of the eyes that will spread toward the head, while there is a sensation or straining in the eyes that feels like sand particles. Euphrasia is also used for eye injuries, especially when a foreign object creates the persistent pain in the eye. It is recommended to use only small doses of euphrasia for eye conditions.

For eye problems, two euphrasia pellets dissolved into a glass of water may be pressed lightly around the eye with a cotton ball twice daily for three days. Further health benefits of euphrasia include it use as liver-protecting and its hypotensive properties.

Sabadilla is a homeopathic remedy for hay fever or other allergies, and worms (not always together). Physical symptoms such as headaches and sore throats start on the left and move to the right side. Symptoms may also appear periodically. The person needing Sabadilla feels chilly, wants warm drinks and may either crave or dislike onions. Symptoms include:

- Nervous, timid, sensitive and imaginative.

- Eyes watering from sensitivity to light.

- Tears with pain.

- Hay fever where the sneezing is the main symptom.

- Hay fever with persistent, violent or sporadic sneezing.

- Hay fever from the odour of flowers or newly mown grass.

- Hay fever that involves the sinuses.

- Hay fever that improves in warm rooms but worsens in open air.

- Itching, tingling and tickling.

- Swallowing caused by a sensation of a lump in the throat.

- Asthma from hay fever.

- Worm infestations.

- Worm infestations that cause twitching or trembling.

- Itching in nose or ears.

The three remedies are sometimes used in combination. Other remedies include natrium muriaticum and pulsatilla. Allergies/ hay fever maybe eased by increasing friendly gut bacteria by regularly consuming fermented foods, miso, live yoghurts and probiotics etc.

For acute and self-limiting complaints, a small dose is usually recommended. Dosing should stop once improvements are noticed. Chronic symptoms or complaints require a course of professional treatment to manage the changes in potencies and remedies that will be required.

Insomnia

<u>Anulom Vilom</u> – This form of pranayama helps to bring about sleep for a restless night.

<u>Avoid caffeine</u> – Try herbal teas as there are so many varieties to choose from or try and cut down on caffeine later in the day.

<u>Bananas</u> boost melatonin and serotonin; these hormones are essential to promote good sleep quality and enhance mood. Bananas contain Tryptophan an amino acid that is essential to promote sleep. Bananas are also rich in magnesium, an important mineral to aid sleep and this mineral is essentially required in most bodily functions.

<u>Cherry</u> – Cherries are highly nutritious and a potent source of anti-oxidants. Cherries reduce inflammation and improve sleep due to the melatonin (sleep hormone), content of the berries. Cherries are one of the only natural foods sources of melatonin.

<u>Fresh Air</u> – Ensure adequate fresh air everyday by going out and enjoy a pollution free environment if possible. Oxygen is very useful at night to induce sleep, leave a bedroom window open at night.

<u>Massage earlobes</u> – Gently massage the earlobes as this can induce sleep. Do not pull or drag the earlobes as this will energise the body and deter sleep.

<u>Grass</u> – Walking on grass barefoot is also extremely beneficial; this practice assists to ground and rebalance the body's magnetic field especially with today lifestyle with electrical, electromagnetic fields (EMF) and radio waves everywhere.

<u>Lavender</u> – This essential Lavender oil in the bath promotes a sense of relaxation. Lavender and chamomile tea can promote a sense of calm and relaxation and are great when used as a sleep aid.

<u>Mindfulness</u> – A state of mindfulness and meditation before bed can induce a restful sleep.

<u>Qigong</u> builds up bone density, slows down the ageing process and improves health. It activates the acupuncture meridians. As well as providing balance, Qigong has many other benefits and can strengthen internal organs, enhance power, reduce stress and promote relaxation,

sleep and healing. Due to its strengthening qualities, Qigong prevents injuries and supports injured parts to heal more quickly.

<u>Serotonin</u> plays an important role in sleep function as it converts to melatonin. A decrease in this neurotransmitter can affect sleep patterns.

<u>Shirodhara</u> is an ancient ayurvedic process. This treatment is performed to ease stress and mental fatigue. This ancient therapy works by pouring a continuous stream of warm oil onto the forehead for half an hour or so; this method acts as an aid to promote calmness and general well-being. This process is proven to improve sleep quality, whether from too much caffeine during the day or restless worries etc. the majority of people have experienced the effects of occasional sleep loss. One single night of lost sleep can cause exhaustion and lethargy. Physical and emotional health can be undermined when sleep quality is constantly compromised. The main solution for decades has been sleep medications, known for their own side effects. Some patients battling insomnia are now looking to more natural holistic therapies, traditional practices and Ayurvedic medicine.

Recent studies investigated the activity in the brains of individuals with insomnia during both waking and sleep states. The results found were people with the sleep disorder showed less powerful alpha-wave activity and more powerful beta-wave activity at all times. In other words, the brains of individuals with chronic insomnia never relaxed.

Shirodhara treatment has been shown to reduce brain waves to the more relaxed alpha state, similar to the effects of meditation. So it stands to reason that this treatment has a beneficial impact on sleep quality. A small study found that this treatment is a successful option "to improve sleep quality and quality of life in persons with sleep problems." Not only was sleep quality improved with this treatment, but better health was experienced. Shirodhara can bring about calm, ease and relaxation to an overactive mind.

<u>Walnuts</u> contain an amino acid called tryptophan that converts into serotonin in the body. Serotonin produces melatonin which aids sleep. Use in moderation, Walnuts like other nuts have been known to cause allergic reactions and taken in excess, these nuts may contribute to a reduction in estrogen production.

Positivity

Positivity is achieved by the regular practice of being positive or optimistic in attitude until it becomes an automatic part of the mindset. Always, focus on the good things it doesn't matter how small. Become aware of your reaction to negative situations and change the negative reactions. Offer positive inspiration to others. Reduce the time spent on social media. Be present and live in the moment as people that practice mindfulness are calmer, are more creative and they are more positive. It is equally essential to have purpose in life, just as it is beneficial to have goals in order to achieve something positive in life. Purpose consists of the central motivating aims in life.

<u>Beliefs</u> – Change negative attitudes to positive, many of the thoughts throughout the day, more often than not tend to be negative. So it is worth being mindful and paying attention to our thoughts and replacing the negative thoughts with positive ones. Instead of telling yourself you are not good enough, state the opposite – you are not inferior to anyone else so do not put yourself down!

<u>Honest Living</u> – Dishonesty brings about guilt and negative emotions. Honesty can bring about a sense of contentment, satisfaction and induce a more positive emotional state. If you are in a position to help someone, you are not losing out in any way but only gaining. This selfless act only assists to support positive moods and emotions. I believe we are all here to help one another. The action to help another is more beneficial and should be done in a selfless manner without expecting anything in return.

<u>Gratitude</u> is a positive emotion that brings positive change to peoples' lives and attitudes. Showing gratitude regularly will create more positive thinking. There are many numerous benefits of genuine gratitude. Try to enjoy life and not worry unnecessarily. It is essential to learn to appreciate your life daily.

Every situation can bring something positive so appreciate every experience and situation. Failures may then become positive aspects of life. Be grateful for everything you have, a home, good health, people who care for you, there's so much to be thankful for; as many do not have this.

You will notice as you shift your focus from the negative thoughts you see things differently and manifest more of the benefits. It is useful to write down the things you appreciate. Many aspects of life are affected by expressing gratitude regularly; emotional health, mental and physical health. Genuine gratitude can bring about the following benefits: - feeling happier with increased optimism; a sense of abundance; contentment; improved self-esteem; a stronger immune system; better sleep; an increased ability to feel grounded; improved relationships and friendships; increased experience of positive emotions; more focus and enjoyment for being in the moment; improvements in psychological and physical health; increased mental strength; improved decision-making; and feeling more empathetic. Therefore it can offer a strong basis for positive change.

It is equally essential to have a purpose in life, just as it is beneficial to have goals in order to achieve something positive in life. Purpose consists of the central motivating aims in life.

Love ♡ yourself – Talk to yourself as if you are talking to a friend. If you were actually talking to a friend, could you get away with the things you are saying to yourself? Never criticise yourself or others. As children we are scolded or told off for something, and as a child in many cases it is a big deal and is misinterpreted as I am not loved! So as adults we carry these experiences but only from a negative point of view. It is important to understand if there are any negative memories, to feel safe and loved in the present! Remind yourself frequently you are always more than good enough and focus on your strengths and positive attributes. Remember you are responsible for your own happiness. Do not depend on others to make you happy or give others the power to make you unhappy.

It also helps to see the good in others, you then are able manifest more of the good qualities you focus on. If you can and are able to help someone do your bit, we are all here to help one another after all and it can really bring benefits and positive changes to a person especially in seeing how lucky we are compared to some and we are able to help someone else in a selfless manner.

Magnesium plays a critical role in brain function and mood. If moods are generally low, or there is a sense of anxiety or panic, it could be due to a deficiency of magnesium.

<u>Mindfulness</u> – It is important to try and remain mindful and in the present as this alleviates stress and worry. As the present moment is probably fine!

<u>Over thinking</u> – It is useful to empty the mind of all thoughts regularly, in order to focus on the present and think logically. Remember for every conscious negative thought state the opposite, positive thought.

<u>Qigong</u> – Builds bone density, slows down the ageing process and improves health. It activates the acupuncture meridians. As well as providing balance, the practice of Qigong helps to strengthen internal organs, enhance power, reduce stress and promote relaxation and healing. Qigong assists with the prevention of injuries and supports injured parts to heal more quickly.

When waking, start the day on a positive note and with a positive attitude, positive intent, clear the barrage of all negative thoughts, fears, grudges and resentments instead try to forgive yourself and others and just say this is a great day and be grateful for the new day. Try to make the most of the day. It might help to go for a walk first thing in the morning to set your-self up on a positive note and experience nature. As you go through the day remain positive and learn to appreciate the day as it unfolds.

Stress

It is important to minimise stress as it is a contributory factor to inflammation. There are many ayurvedic herbs, supplements and treatments that help manage stress. The herbs are known as adaptogens; thought to have health benefits and act as aids in stress reduction. Herbs such as Ashwaghanda, Bhringraj, Brahmi, Tulsi, Maca, and yoga and ayurvedic treatments as mentioned below all support stress reduction and the management of stress.

Good breathing is a major component of good health. Long deep breaths and long exhales are beneficial in getting enough oxygen into the body and releasing carbon dioxide properly. Proper breathing is useful in anxiety and stress reduction. Breathing through the nose is more beneficial than breathing through the mouth.

For a calming effect rub Brahmi/Bhringraj oil into scalp and feet before bed. Mindfulness staying present in the moment is beneficial for calmness and a regular head and body massage can be extremely beneficial.

Meditation is a great way to reduce stress and promote calm. As meditation regulates the sympathetic and autonomic nervous systems and so controls our responses during sudden stress encounters.

Ensure a twenty-minute activity each day. Brisk walking, yoga, dancing or even running are very beneficial just to get the heart pumping, circulation and hormones moving as well as provide a release for stress.

Walking on grass barefoot is also extremely beneficial, especially having contact with earth. It helps to ground and rebalance the body's magnetic field especially with today's hectic lifestyle with electrical, Emf (electromagnetic fields), radio waves everywhere. The contact with the soil daily is extremely beneficial and so too is being outdoors in nature.

<u>Nasya</u> — This ayurvedic remedy traditionally assists the nervous system and corresponding issues. Medicated oils, ghee or coconut oil nurture and nourish the nerves of the brain and head. Nasya

may prove very beneficial for the ears, migraines, headaches, sinus problems, the nose, general health and stress due to its affects on the nervous system. It protects against allergens such as pollen as it lubricates the nasal passages. This process works by inserting a few drops of medicated oils or ghee into the nostrils whilst the head is tilted.

Shirodhara is an ancient ayurvedic treatment designed to ease physiological stress and mental fatigue. It is a simple ancient therapy whereby a stream of warm oil is poured onto the forehead for a half an hour to promote calmness and general well-being. Shirodhara has the effect of reducing the brainwaves to a more relaxed alpha state. Shirodhara as an ideal treatment for reducing high levels of mental stress as it induces calmness, promotes tranquility, and facilitates relaxation. The steady pour of warm oil encourages the relaxation response where the body enters deep relaxation, stress hormones decline while hyper-alert brain patterns (beta waves) transition into relaxed-alert ones (alpha waves). The relaxation response is the body's way of turning on the parasympathetic nervous system, that part of the nervous system which conserves energy, slows heart rate, and relaxes muscles.

Ujjayi pranayama – This form of pranayama which practiced correctly brings about a sense of calm.

Walks in nature and generally being around nature are great ways to support stress reduction. Breathing properly and taking time out all have very positive effects on stress reduction. Relaxation modalities such as yoga, meditation and mindfulness, Epsom salt baths are very beneficial in the management of stress.

Weight loss

<u>Almonds</u> are rich in nutrients. These nuts are high in anti-oxidants and vitamin E. Almonds reduce blood sugar and lower cholesterol. Other benefits of almonds include their ability to satisfy hunger and promote weight loss.

<u>Bananas</u> are satiating; have the capability to reduce the appetite as well as ease food cravings due to their ability to regulate blood sugar.

<u>Eat a healthy diet</u> avoid refined sugar and fried foods or moderate the intake of these foods. Eat more fresh fruit and vegetables and healthy fats. Eat meals on time, avoid snacking in between meals, and also eat a healthy portion size this will help with gradual weight loss use a plate as a guide. Do not miss meals as hormones become imbalanced and cravings for junk food occur. Daily exercise even brisk walking approximately 20 minutes per day helps to define and tone the body. Try to be active as it's really important and integral to weight loss. Take up a new activity; ensure a good night's sleep to help with moods to reduce food cravings.

<u>Bamboo shoot</u> is nutritionally dense, due this composition it reduces unhealthy food cravings in the body. Similarly the same is said for blackstrap molasses due the content of vitamins and minerals in natural whole food source.

<u>Matcha Green Tea</u> – As green tea normally reduces fat in the body, matcha tea being a concentration of green tea can aid in weight loss quite quickly.

<u>Saffron</u> – This plant is rich in anti-oxidants. The flavonoids in saffron protect the body against fungal infections. Due to its ability to produce serotonin, it can improve mood and decrease depression; therefore it acts as an aid to curb the appetite, reduce cravings, aid weight loss and aid hormonal balance to ease menstruation symptoms.

<u>Sugar Cravings</u> – This may indicate a chromium deficiency. Blackstrap molasses are a rich source of chromium. Sugar cravings are reduced

by eating a balanced meal including carbohydrates, protein etc, on a timely basis and by not skipping meals. Nettle leafs contain compounds that enhance glucose absorption; these compounds act like insulin; they can improve blood sugar levels as a result. This is a major benefit for hormonal health because symptoms and conditions like PCOS and weight gain are tied to elevated blood sugar levels.

Women's Health

Evidence suggests that women are more prone than men to experience anxiety, depression, and somatic complaints – physical symptoms that cannot be explained medically. Depression is most commonly experienced in women. Sometimes the low moods can be brought about by poor diet, lack of exercise, hormonal irregularities, changes in lifestyle and stress which can all be contributing factors. Essentially it is important to address these issues. Eating a balanced diet, regular exercise, stress reduction techniques, and in some instances, herbal remedies may be essential in alleviating these issues. Some herbal remedies are mentioned as below are discussed in detail for women's issues.

<u>Agnus-castus</u> (Vitex/Chasteberry) is a plant used in herbal medicine. It is often used to remedy women's health problems as it may improve the symptoms of PMS and assist with the management of menopausal symptoms.

As in the case of Maca, this plant has been cultivated for over 2000 years. It is widely used in Peru.

The benefits of maca powder for women are: to relieve the problems associated with menopause and menstruation; boost fertility in women; lower blood pressure, and balance hormones. This nutritional compound has an ability to boost energy levels; improve bone health, improve sexual health and function. It also assists with the maintenance of a healthy immune system, improvement of skin health, and to build stamina. The root of the Maca plant is used mainly.

During menopause there is a natural decline in estrogen that occurs throughout this time; this can cause a range of unpleasant symptoms. Some of which include hot flashes, mood swings, sleep disruption problems and irritability.

Studies have shown that by taking maca powder daily, (a dosage of 1-1.5 tsp); great benefits for hormone regularity were seen. The minimum suggested treatment time is 6-12 weeks. Generally a break is recommended after this time, a week or so. Beyond this, maca may be consumed daily and regularly to maintain positive benefits.

Maca should be considered as "non-hormonal" in nature. Instead, maca should be viewed as exhibiting hormone-regulatory properties across a wide range of age groups of women and men. It seems to induce the hormone balance that is needed for a given individual, specific to a person's gender, age and metabolic stage.

<u>Raspberry Leaf</u> – Many women suffer from hormonal issues that make it difficult for them to conceive. Raspberry leaf tea has been shown to increase fertility in some of these women due to its ability to balance hormone levels.

Further research has been completed, confirming Raspberry Leaf benefits for menstruation.

Raspberry leaf tea is known to ease menstrual discomfort in women. It is known to relieve heavy bleeding, cramping, headaches and stomach discomfort. The ingredient fragarine is known to help tone and tighten the pelvic region muscles as well as ease cramps caused by the spasms of the muscles in this area. Tannins are believed to strengthen the uterus, mitigating heavy and irregular menstrual bleeding; this herbal remedy is thought to tone the muscles of the uterus (womb), to support its work during labour and to assist labour progress at a steady pace. Caffeine/tea should not be consumed during pregnancy; commonly some women consume it only after the third trimester (32 weeks onwards).

<u>Shatavari</u> is considered a supreme tonic and hormonal regulator for women's health. It is known to support women through every stage of life. Shatavari's main constituents are mainly its use as an estrogen regulator. This modulation helps to regulate menstrual cycles, manage PMS symptoms, alleviate menstrual cramps and control the amount of blood lost. Shatavari greatly aids fluid retention and may be helpful with the uncomfortable bloating before a period. This versatile herb is useful to women with fertility issues as it lines and protects the cervix. It can protect against miscarriage. Due to its oily, heavy nature, Shatavari nourishes the female reproductive system from within to relieve menopausal symptoms such as vaginal dryness, hot flashes and insomnia. This phytoestrogen-rich herb naturally helps to balance the hormones responsible for many of the more unpleasant symptoms during this change in life. Shatavari also stimulates and balances the mood enhancing hormones; endorphins, serotonin and dopamine - so mood swings are reduced; feelings of irritability and menopause induced depression are also reduced. It also acts as an aphrodisiac.

A to Z of General Remedies

This book is not intended to be a substitute for medical advice I recommend you seek independent medical advice before following any of the teachings or suggestions in this book. The author and publisher accept no liability or responsibility in the case of personal injury.

Any remedies, supplements and treatments recommended are subject to the manufacturers recommendations if unsure please contact your medical professional or the manufacturer.

Acupressure – This is a less invasive method than acupuncture for treatment and release of blockages associated with many ailments and pain. Symptoms may be eased by applying localised pressure on various points depending upon the ailment. Speak with an acupressure practitioner for further advice.

ADHD – Lavender oils/sesame oils and Epsom salt baths can provide relief from the hyperactivity associated with ADHD. Shirodhara is a calming and stress reducing therapy and has proven beneficial in reducing the symptoms of ADHD. Cranial sacral therapy has proven valuable for relieving the symptoms of ADHD in children. Other methods to ease symptoms of ADHD include - Regular walks in nature and walking barefoot on grass induces a sense of calm. Meditation promotes focus and concentration and with regular practice it may also reduce hyperactivity. The treatments mentioned also have beneficial effects for people suffering with arthritis and other auto-immune disorders. An alkaline diet can be especially useful for the latter cases and for general health.

Agnus Castus – This herb is a natural source of progesterone; it assists to balance the ratio of estrogen to progesterone, so is used to regulate the menstrual cycle. It can be especially useful for fertility issues, PMS and to reverse PCOS.

Allergies – A saline solution of water and salt poured through the nostrils can be very effective to treat sinus, runny nose and seasonal allergies. This method used long-term can really alleviate allergies. Cinnamon and honey taken in the morning as a natural antibiotic can clear bacteria, fungus and viral infections. Refer to the Hay fever section for more information on allergies.

<u>Aloe Vera</u> – This succulent plant is normally used as a digestive aid as it works to balance stomach acids. It has laxative qualities and is beneficial for cases of constipation and IBS. Aloe Vera contains a huge array of vitamins A, B2, B3 and B6, C and E as well as an abundance of minerals. It is rich in Choline and Folic Acid, all of which allow the skin to regenerate and stay healthy. This plant supports the maintenance of strong healthy hair and a healthy scalp. It eases burns, sunburn and may be used as an after sun moisturiser.

<u>Amla</u> – Amla is beneficial for the immune system and provides rejuvenation of the skin and hair. It contains high levels of Vitamin C and other anti-oxidants. It slows down the ageing process, it can treat throat infections and improve heart health and reduce blood sugar levels. Regular consumption of this fruit provides major health benefits. Also known as Amalaki: amla assists many issues such as digestive problems, jaundice, diabetes, colic, peptic ulcers, anaemia, nausea, vomiting, skin disease, cardiac problems, cold, fever, hair problems, nerve issues and gum and teeth health.

<u>Anti-oxidants</u> are substances that inhibit oxidation, especially used to counteract the deterioration of stored food products. "Anti-oxidant" as mentioned is a general term for any compound that can counteract unstable molecules called free radicals that damage DNA, cell membranes, and other parts of cells. Vitamin C or E serve as anti-oxidants that remove potentially damaging oxidizing agents in a living organism. Generally, they assist with the defence of the cells from the damage caused by potentially harmful molecules known as free radicals, as when free radicals accumulate, they can cause a state known as oxidative stress. This may damage your DNA and also damage other important structures in your cells. As suggested some vitamins and minerals — including vitamins C and E and the minerals copper, zinc, and selenium — all function as anti-oxidants, in addition to other vital roles. Some other anti oxidants are listed as follows together with their functions; Beta carotene as this supports the immune system, vision and healthy skin; Lycopene, protects organisms from excessive light damage, Lutein which is great for eyes; Quercetin as an anti-inflammatory, improves allergies, lowers blood pressure; Rutin improves circulation, prevents blood clots, lowers pain.

<u>Anulom Vilom</u> – Experts believe Anulom Vilom pranayama may have an immediate calming effect; a great way to start the day. The benefits include great health and positivity. It is one of the most satisfying breathing exercises practiced by many people. It can have a positive effect on the lungs, nasal pipe, esophagus, and the trachea. Alternate nostril breathing has been of special significance in Yoga as it can enhance the respiratory system.

A recent study on a group of people that performed Anulom Vilom Pranayama daily, concluded there was also highly significant improvement of cognition, general well-being and reduced anxiety. It improves concentration and the ability to focus. Studies explain how this yoga may be practiced by children to support them to become calm and focused.

Breathing deeply with more awareness releases the tension surrounding the heart muscles and tissues. This allows blood pressure levels to normalise. By performing this breathing activity daily heart beat rate per minute can improve.

Be very careful when performing yoga on an empty stomach. Remember, always to have a glass of warm water when you wake up to cleanse the system and remember it is important to hydrate before yoga practice and breathing exercises.

<u>Apple cider Vinegar</u> use in the diet offers many health benefits. Some of these benefits include weight loss, lower cholesterol, lower blood sugar as well as improvements in diabetes conditions. Apple cider vinegar diluted and applied to the scalp may reduce hair-loss as it restores the ph balance of the scalp. Organic raw unfiltered acv contains proteins and enzymes and probiotic bacteria called the mother these are responsible for healthy acv and general gut health. Apple cider vinegar helps with arthritis conditions, acv is alkaline in nature.

<u>Argan oil</u> has moisturizing properties that help maintain skin elasticity while preventing moisture loss, as this contributes to aging of the skin. This oil makes the skin softer while limiting the appearance of stretch marks and is also nourishing for the hair.

<u>Arnica</u> – A homeopathic remedy useful for treating shock. Arnica in the form of a gel applied to bruises, sprains, muscle pain for chronic conditions and arthritis relieves the pain due to its

anti-inflammatory properties. Skin benefits are also noticed with regular use of arnica gel.

<u>Arthritis and other care uses</u> – Arthritis is a condition causing the swelling and tenderness of one or more joints; main symptoms of arthritis are joint pain and stiffness, which typically worsen with age. The most common types of arthritis are osteoarthritis; this causes cartilage to breakdown and rheumatoid arthritis is when the immune system attacks the joints.

Treatments vary depending on the type of arthritis. The main goals of arthritis treatments are to reduce symptoms and improve quality of life. Urgent medical attention is usually recommended in severe cases by healthcare providers and arthritis can last several years or be temporary.

Many times the symptoms of arthritis aren't fully controlled by conventional medicine. There are many alternative medicines. Chiropractors may assist with the relief of some of the symptoms of arthritis. Physiotherapists use acupuncture. Panchakarma is an ayurvedic treatment – a way of cleansing the body to restore immunity; it is a holistic way of getting to the root cause of the issue much like Traditional Chinese Medicine. The practice of self-care and stress relief is very important for managing chronic diseases like arthritis.

Regularly soaking in Epsom or mineral salt baths provides considerable relief and healing for arthritis sufferers due to the magnesium and mineral content of these salts and a reduction to inflammation markers. The heat from the warm water is very soothing to stiff joints. The benefits of warm water include muscle relaxation, improved joint mobility, and reduced pain. Various healing modalities are mentioned throughout which are useful for pain and stress relief -yoga and meditation are especially useful to ease these symptoms. Some use apple cider vinegar, ginger, lemons and turmeric. An essential component to ease arthritis symptoms involves a change of diet to include a more alkaline diet, a diet rich in essential nutrients and an anti-inflammatory diet.

<u>Ashwagandha</u> – An ayurvedic extract used to ease anxiety and stress. This adaptogen herb works on the adrenal glands; to reduce and regulate the cortisol hormone which is responsible for stress.

Ashwaghanda supports a healthy nervous system due to its nourishing and energising effects. It assists with thyroid related problems, particularly hypothyroidism as it impacts the pituitary gland and this in turn increases T4 hormones. Summary T4, or thyroxine, is a type of thyroid hormone that regulates metabolism. It also plays an important role in digestion, muscle function, and bone health. Although T4 levels differ from person to person, they usually exist within a normal range. This should not be taken with other thyroid medication as it may cause an imbalance in the thyroid.

Asthma – Chyawanprash is an ancient ayurvedic herbal jam; known to possess the ability to balance the water in the lungs. There are many other countless health benefits of using this product known to help in the reversal of the ageing process, restore muscle and bone density. Tiger milk mushroom helps soothe respiratory inflammation, eases breathing and relieves asthma.

Ayurvedic massages consist of different ayurvedic massage therapies focusing on the specific disease or parts of the body. Each of these massages comes with a range of physical and mental benefits. They are mostly carried out to stimulate and relax the muscles and joints in the body so that the herbs and oils can work deeply to eradicate the disease.

Bad Cholesterol – A favourable way to reduce bad cholesterol is by eating porridge regularly. Oats contain soluble fibre that works on reducing bad cholesterol. Turmeric and bamboo shoot have similar properties so work in the same way to decrease cholesterol.

Bala – This ayurvedic herb known as sida cordifolia is mainly used to treat inflammatory conditions. The bark, flower, root and stem are all used. Bala imparts inner strength. Due to its potency, only a very small amount is recommended for internal use. This herb is used by athletes for strength training. Bala is a nourishing tonic, especially for nervous conditions. According to ayurvedic uses, it balances all the individual constitutions. This herb is beneficial in treating immune related conditions; urinary problems such as stones; Bala is proven to be effective in the treatment of sinus and other infections. It is Rasayana and useful for all kinds of rheumatic disorders. This health tonic offers rejuvenating, anti-inflammatory, libido-enhancing and fat-burning properties. Sida cordifolia or Bala has analgesic, aphrodisiac, demulcent, diuretic, nervine, rejuvenative, stimulant, tonic and curative properties. External application of this herb is used to reduce arthritis pain and ease joint stiffness. Oil prepared from this herb is used to treat spondylitis and paralysis. This herb assists in the absorption of water and nutrients from the intestine and is very good for irritable bowel syndrome. It is used to reduce chest congestion, bronchitis and asthma. Bala has proven beneficial for the treatment of blood and bile disorders.

Although excessive use can cause serious contra indications such as an increase in blood pressure, stress, insomnia, nervousness and more serious consequences.

Bamboo shoot is rich in silica; this converts to collagen and nourishes thinning hair, skin and muscles. It helps with hair loss, strengthens weak and brittle nails, bones, muscles and skin. This extract helps support the vascular system, reduce cholesterol, and prevent heart disease. It also supports the nervous system, with its high concentration of vitamins, minerals and amino acids. Bamboo plant also promotes healthy digestion and glandular system health.

Bananas are a source of many vitamins and minerals. These fruits are beneficial to health and are rich in vitamin B6, biotin, melatonin, serotonin as well as an amino acid called tryptophan that assists to promote better sleep. The magnesium in bananas can ease anxiety and stress. Bananas are satiating and are able to reduce the appetite and ease food cravings due to their ability to regulate blood sugar. They are good for bone health and aid regular bowel movements.

Beliefs – Change negative attitudes to positive, many of the thoughts throughout the day, more often than not tend to be negative. So it is worth being mindful and paying attention to our thoughts and replacing the negative thoughts with positive thoughts. Instead of telling yourself you cannot do this, state the opposite – I can do this! Silence the inner critic.

Bhumyamalaki – This ayurvedic herb is mainly used to repair the liver and is also a good liver cleanser. It is also known as the stonebreaker and is used to ease the symptoms associated with kidney stones, as well as aid liver and kidney function.

<u>Bibhitaki</u> – An ayurvedic herb, known to ease digestive problems, diarrhea, dyspepsia, hemorrhoids, hepatitis, bronchitis, fevers, coughs, asthma, eye disease, hair problems, and scorpion sting.

<u>Black strap molasses</u> contain calcium, iron, magnesium and many other nutrients and anti-oxidants. It is the beneficial part of sugar that is usually disposed of. Sugar cravings are reduced when taken regularly as it contains chromium as it stabilises blood sugar levels. Other benefits include reduced menstrual problems. This syrup acts as a good blood promoter and offers beneficial qualities for bone, skin, muscle/hair health and assists stress reduction. Some have seen molasses dissolve blood clots in the legs when taken long-term. It may be used as a replacement for sugar, even taken as a drink and be used in cooking/baking. Due to the presence of lots of beneficial minerals it is also very useful in reducing stress and anxiety.

<u>Breathing</u> – Good breathing is a major component of good health. Long deep breaths and long exhales are beneficial in allowing enough oxygen into the body and releasing carbon dioxide properly. Proper breathing is useful in stress reduction. Breathing through the nose is more beneficial than breathing through the mouth. Breathing in through the left nostril will access the right hemisphere of the brain or emotional side or creative part of the brain. Breathing in through the right nostril, will access the left hemisphere of the brain, the part that deals with logic. Unconscious alternating of the nostrils for breathing happens automatically throughout day.

<u>Bhringraj Powder</u> – This ayurvedic herb supports healthy hair growth and is normally used as a cure for baldness: Bhringraj helps to boost blood circulation in the scalp region and follicles, this in turn results in more nutrients supplied to the root of the hair.

Bhringraj is a great herb used to treat dandruff and scalp itchiness: various types of dandruff mostly occur due to extreme dry scalp and humidity in the atmospheric air.

It is beneficial for the liver and is used to aid regeneration of the liver: The liver is primarily associated with the metabolism activity of the body and Bhringraj is used to improve metabolism as it has amazing digestive properties.

Bhringraj has exceptional properties which are useful to alleviate indigestion issues, constipation and appetite loss. Due to its high magnesium content Bhringraj can prevent headaches, memory loss and migraines, and may promote muscle relaxation, sleep and improve mood.

Bhringraj is used to relieve body pain: The juice extracted from fresh Bhringraj leaves is beneficial in relieving body pain, swelling issues and inflammation.

Due to its calming effect on the adrenal glands, the intake of this herb or application of oil has a positive effect on the nervous system. As a result of this affect Bhringraj can ease or prevent nervous system disorders as well as calm palpitations of the heart; with regular use bhringraj improves memory power and reduces aggressiveness.

<u>Burdock root</u> is closely related to the daisy and sunflower family. Medicinally, the whole plant is edible. The root is most often used for its health benefits, as Burdock root has a long tapering root. This herb has been used for centuries in Ayurvedic, Traditional Chinese Medicine and western herbal medicine. It can be harvested fresh from the ground or bought dried.

The key benefits of burdock root include:

- It is one of the best herbs for stimulating lymphatic drainage and relieving congestion. This herb promotes overall immune system health, as the lymphatic system or the inner drainage system of the body which is a very important part of the immune system. A healthy lymphatic system helps move toxins out of the body as well as carrying lymph (infection-fighting white blood cells) throughout the body. When this system becomes congested swollen lymph nodes occur. Burdock root is one of the safer herbs without side effects and maybe be drank as tea throughout the day to cleanse the lymphatic system.

- This herb has also shown benefits for treating and preventing diabetes. A few recent studies indicate that burdock can help with insulin levels, lower bad cholesterol levels, and raise good cholesterol levels. Its anti-oxidant content also appears to have a favorable effect on symptoms of diabetes. In addition, burdock root contains a prebiotic fiber called inulin. Inulin can help improve digestion and naturally lower blood sugar levels.

- Like other parts of the body, the bloodstream can also become burdened with toxins; burdock root has traditionally been considered a blood purifier and is still used for this purpose today. It can remove toxins from the bloodstream and also improves circulation, which in turn improves the appearance of skin. Burdock root is perhaps most used in herbal medicine because of its benefits for the skin. It is considered one of the best herbs for the skin and can be used internally or externally. Burdock's ability to purify the blood is one reason it is so beneficial for the skin. Toxins in the body and in the bloodstream can contribute to skin problems like eczema and psoriasis. Taking burdock root as a tea or tincture will help clear out those toxins. Burdock root is also considered a cooling herb and helps to cool "hot," inflammatory skin conditions like acne and eczema. It can be taken internally for this purpose or use externally as a wash. Burdock also has a high anti-oxidant content which benefits skin and improves signs of aging, including wrinkles.

<u>Calendula</u> is a great bitter herb that can stimulate the liver, digestion, and lymphatic system. Many herbalists also recommend calendula for repairing the gut, which will greatly improve the body's natural detoxification system. It is also great for calming skin conditions and is used in natural skin creams for babies. Calendula flowers can be used fresh or dried, usually as a tea to support internal health. The tea will be very bitter but is also very useful.

<u>Calm</u> – For a calming effect rub Brahmi/Bhringraj oil into scalp and feet before bed. Mindfulness staying present in the moment is beneficial for calmness. Taking deep long breaths, meditation and being close to nature all induce a sense of calm.

<u>Candida</u> is a type of yeast that is found in the digestive tract. When the level of Candida in the gut becomes too high, it can cause an infection known as Candida overgrowth which can cause a variety of uncomfortable symptoms. <u>Candida overgrowth</u>; this is a chronic health condition that affects many people. It can appear on various parts of

the body but is often related to an imbalance in the gut flora. Until that gut imbalance is addressed, the symptoms of Candida may be difficult to treat. Vitality will return once this overgrowth is addressed, you will feel more energetic and clarity of mind will be restored.

As many conditions may be caused by candida. It may not be obvious and things like mood swings, a weak immune system, brain fog, chronic fatigue, digestive problems, food sensitivities, joint pain, oral thrush, recurring sinus and fungal infections, fatigue, skin infections, and many more may all be symptoms of a candida overgrowth. This overgrowth may be the result of overuse of antibiotics, diabetes, diet, chemical exposure, chronic stress, hormonal imbalance, mercury fillings and sugar to name a few.

Most of the time natural remedies can stop candida overgrowth. For stubborn candida overgrowth there will be a need to consult a holistic and medical professional.

Candida yeast overgrowth can be restricted with the following natural methods. It takes time but it can completely clean your system from the overgrowth with persistence. Remember that treating Candida overgrowth in its early stages has several long-term health benefits. If it remains untreated, it can confuse diagnosis and cure in most cases, as its symptoms mimic many other diseases.

There are three simple stages that may be used as an approach to cure candida overgrowth.

- <u>Stop The Yeast Overgrowth</u> - In order to restrict the overgrowth you have to stop feeding the candida. Eliminate all sugars that feed candida from the diet, which means a switch to a low-carbohydrate diet. Give up all sources of sugar including candies, deserts, alcohol, and refined flours. Move to whole grains, fruits, beans, etc.

- <u>Rebuild the Good Gut Bacteria</u> - Consume plant based foods, vegetables, grains and beans (pre-biotics), as they have been shown to feed a positive gut environment. Fibre directly feeds gut bacteria, as it is broken down in the large intestine where most of our gut micro biota are housed.

- <u>Ensure bacteria does not move into the Bloodstream</u> - Eliminate all the foods and minimise caffeine and eliminate alcohol, refined foods, starchy foods and added sugars that can harm the GI tract so that the yeast doesn't move to the rest of the body. Healing the gut is a very important part of that process to get rid of candida overgrowth from the system. Include healthy proteins and probiotics in the diet.

There are several simple home remedies that can help treat Candida overgrowth. Natural treatments can work better. Colloidial Silver is used to treat fungal infections such as athlete's foot.

- ACV is useful for the treatment of oral thrush; thus another good treatment for Candida. Mix 3 teaspoons of apple cider vinegar in a glass of water. Gargle vigorously with the solution. Ensure that the solution is not swallowed. Don't rinse it. This will leave traces of apple cider vinegar on the affected area and cure candida overgrowth.

- Due to its many health benefits, Coconut oil has received prominence recently; this is owing to some of it properties as it contains many medium-chain fatty acids such as lauric, caprylic, and capric acid which have anti-fungal and antimicrobial capabilities. These fatty acids can kill candida. To clear candidiasis take one teaspoon of unrefined virgin coconut oil daily.

- Cranberries are also very beneficial for heart health. Cranberries contain an anti-fungal compound called arbutin to kill Candida albicans. Taking them regularly can help get rid of the candida overgrowth within a short time. Buy non-sweetened fresh cranberry juice. Drink a glass of cranberry juice twice a day for a couple of weeks to get fast results.

- Garlic is a natural anti-fungal and anti-bacterial agent. It has many sulfur-containing compounds to help fight Candida infections.

- Oregano oil can be used to get rid of candidiasis due to its anti-fungal and antimicrobial capabilities. A compound called carvacrol in oregano oil stops the growth of Candida yeast. Scientific studies have also found that the oil's agents can be effective in treating as well as preventing candidiasis. Ensure that you don't consume too much oregano oil. 2-3 drops are enough. You can add in a glass of water and drink the mix.

You can drink it twice daily for a few days, Oregano oil also comes in capsule forms.

- Tea Tree is useful in treating oral thrush, (candida overgrowth). Add 10 drops of Tree tea oil to a glass of water. Take a mouthful from the glass and gargle for a minute. Repeat it until the entire solution is finished. Let the mixture touch all internal surfaces of the mouth while gargling, also ensure that you don't swallow the solution. Twice a day is beneficial— one just after waking up and the other before going to bed.

- An excellent treatment for Candida is Yogurt. It contains probiotics that repair candidiasis. Yogurt keeps the candida in check as the live Lactobacillus acidophilus culture produces lactic acid which stops candida overgrowth. It can be applied on all affected areas of the outer skin. It may be left on the area for an hour and wash it completely and dry it. It not only cures Candida from the skin but also reduces itching and weeping.

All remedies may take a few months to cure candida. There may be a die off period in which case you may feel worse before feeling better. In addition to the use of remedies to cure candida, the use of preventative methods may assist with the discouragement of candida yeast infection.

Candida fungus can flourish in damp environments and the body provides many opportunities to store moisture such as the armpits, etc. These areas should be kept dry. An essential part as well is to maintain a healthy immune system as a lack of nutrients, dehydration, inadequate sleep, stress, toxins and chemicals etc may impact and weaken immunity. The excessive use of antibiotics develops resistance to various conditions due to developing a resistance to antibiotics; the microbes cause other complications such as candida overgrowth. Antibiotics should be used with discretion. In addition to killing bad bacteria antibiotics also kill so many other good bacteria that are required for good gut health as a result this causes the proportion of the Candida albicans to increase which results in candida overgrowth and infection. Taking probiotics may address this issue when taking anti-biotics, but take them a few hours apart.

The current fast lifestyle of fast foods and overindulgence in carbohydrates increases blood sugar levels. Candida albicans thrive on sugar, so avoid sugar. Reduce the consumption of carbohydrates which produce extra sugar in the body during the treatment of candida overgrowth.

The Immune system may be suppressed by the toxic substances in drugs, medicines, birth control pills, vaccines, chemicals, gm foods and fluoridated water. Maintain proper hygiene. Remain hydrated by drinking lots of water, get sufficient rest, exercise regularly and eat nutritious food, to prevent candida overgrowth to also assist overall health.

<u>Cardamom</u> is a spice that has been used for centuries both in cooking and as a medicine. Originally this seed is a common ingredient in Indian, Middle Eastern and Arabic foods. People may also take cardamom as a supplement for its health benefits. Cardamom contains phytochemicals that have anti-inflammatory and anti-bacterial properties. Other health benefits of Cardamom include:

- Its anti-microbial abilities.

- It's anti-oxidant and diuretic properties may lower blood pressure.

- Its anti-inflammatory effects that may protect from chronic diseases.

- Cardamom assists digestive issues, including ulcers.

- It may treat bad breath and prevent cavities

- Cardamom improves hemoglobin and insulin levels.

- Cardamom improves heart health.

<u>Castor oil</u> – Applying drops of this oil in the eyes at night lubricates the eyes and treats dry eyes. The properties of this oil include its anti-inflammatory and anti-bacterial abilities as it rids the eyes of infective bacteria. In India, castor oil was the ancient treatment used for cataracts long before the advent of medicine. This oil was used to dissolve cataracts, before further progression to the late stage of cataracts. Cataracts occur when there is a build- up of the protein structure/film that forms clumps on the lens and disrupts vision. With regular use the properties of Castor oil repair the lens to restore the eyesight and dissolve the protein film that had formed on the lens over time.

Castor oil also promotes healthier cell growth in the eye and restores lost moisture in the eyes as it contains ricinoleic acid an omega 3 fatty acid that assists with collagen production and skin renewal. The key nutrients in castor oil are beneficial for dry eyes. Castor oil use promotes collagen production. Castor oil used on the scalp and hair shows visible improvements for thin, dry and frizzy hair.

Cayenne has many health benefits mainly attributed to the ingredient capsaicin. The pepper contains vitamin A, C, vitamin B6, vitamin E, potassium, manganese, and flavonoids. Open wounds or breaks in the skin should not be exposed to capsaicin. It provides beneficial plant compounds that are useful for heart health. It improves digestion and helps to support a healthy weight. Capsaicin is known to ease pain, clear congestion and headaches. Capsaicin is also used in topical form to treat pain. Creams made from the potent spice can be rubbed on the sore areas to treat arthritis pain.

Celery Juice – There are many benefits of juicing generally, due to the nutrients being more readily available. Celery Juice on its own is especially very beneficial as it is nutrient dense; with long-term consumption, celery Juice may reduce inflammation, aid gut health, reduce pathogens and act as a great liver detoxifier. It is packed full of vitamins and minerals and is able to balance electrolytes in the body. This juice assists cell renewal as it contains mineral salts and silica.

Cherry – Are highly nutritious and a potent source of anti-oxidants. Cherries reduce inflammation in the body as well act to aid sleep. Cherries are particularly good at reducing symptoms of gout. Other benefits of cherries are that they possess the nutritional potential to slow down ageing and ward off chronic illness.

Chlorella – These algae have many anti-oxidant benefits that assist in detoxification of the body and enhance the immune function. Chlorella contains lots of nutrients; is known to regulate blood sugar and reduce high blood pressure. It binds to heavy metals to rid the body of these toxins. Chlorella is known as a super-food due to its nutritionally dense composition.

Chyawanprash is beneficial for the treatment of colds and flu. Chyawanprash assists the body in purification of the blood and elimination of harmful toxins. It supports the healthy function of the heart and respiratory system as it balances the fluid in the lungs. Chyawanprash can improve digestive health; rejuvenate all tissues in the body, improve the complexion and promote healthy bone and muscle mass.

<u>Cinnamon</u> (Ceylon cinnamon) a substance packed with potent medicinal qualities, a good blood thinner, best known to regulate blood sugar and aid diabetes 2. It is well known as an anti-inflammatory and may prevent the risk of heart disease. Cinnamon contains more anti-oxidant compounds than garlic and oregano. Cinnamon has anti-bacterial, anti-viral and anti-fungal properties; when taken with honey it pacifies viral infections and colds. Cassia cinnamon contains the compound coumarin which can be toxic to the liver.

<u>Cloves</u> are antimicrobial; used in mouth wash they are able to improve gum health as they reduce plaque and bacteria. Cloves very nutritious and rich in healthy antioxidants; they may improve liver health due to the compound eugenol. Cloves should only be consumed in small quantities as cloves may cause excess bleeding. Cloves should be avoided for those taking blood thinning medication.

<u>Colloidial Silver</u> is used as an antibiotic as it has anti-microbial effects. It can kill viruses, fungal infections and bacteria. It is a viable alternative to treat various anti-fungal candida infections. It can stimulate healing in skin and soft tissue and inflammation. It should be used in moderation and short-term as it can cause discolouration of bodily tissues especially when the product has been processed manually.

<u>Colon cleanse</u> is beneficial as it supports the body in the elimination of old stored food waste, pathogens and toxins with the purpose to get health back on track.

<u>Constipation</u> – Treat constipation by drinking two glasses of warm water first thing in the morning. Drinking aloe vera juice and prune juice are also beneficial with the relief of constipation. Eating figs and taking magnesium before bed improve bowel function. There is an acupressure point measuring three fingers width on both sides of the belly button; this is useful as by gently pressing these points on both sides of the belly button so the bowel movements are managed with ease.

<u>Copper</u> stimulates the brain, prevents premature ageing, improves functions of the thyroid gland, assists the body in the production of healthy blood cells and supports the maintenance of bones, improved immune functions and iron absorption. It is naturally occurring in nuts, seeds, leafy green vegetables, turmeric and dark chocolate.

<u>Coriander</u> – The anti-oxidants in coriander prevent eyes diseases and eye related problems, it is anti-bacterial and anti-fungal and a good treatment of conjunctivitis. Coriander has the ability to normalise blood sugar; promote healthy liver function and maintain cardiovascular health. It works as a natural deodorant and also a cooling herb for excess heat in the body.

<u>Cough & Cold & Sore Throat</u> – Taking a mixture of Cinnamon and honey is very beneficial to fight off the bacteria and bugs that cause common cold and virus due to the natural anti-biotic abilities when combined. Ginger and lemon are very good at alkalising the body; infection can only flourish in an acidic environment. Chyawanprash is good at stimulating the body's immune response to infection.

<u>Cranial-sacral Therapy</u> – It is an alternative treatment using the hands to gently work on the body; to assist the body with the release of traumas, relief of pain, tension as well as many other supportive benefits for a lot of ailments especially in children. Basically a gentle compression is applied in the sacrum, bones of the head and throughout the body. It supports the body's ability to balance, heal and restore itself, and it is promoted as a cure for a variety of health issues.

It works by using subtle manipulations that affect the circulation and pressure of cerebrospinal fluid and it is a very calming and relaxation promoting therapy.

<u>Cumin</u> – It contains properties that ward off infections and prevent anaemia. Cumin has become a subject of medical research as there are a wide range of health benefits to using it as well as vitamins, iron, copper, calcium and zinc. Cumin can be a little heating on the body when consumed in excess.

<u>Daily exercise</u> – Ensure a twenty-minute activity each day. Brisk walking, yoga, dancing and even running are good ways to get the heart pumping. Regular physical activity improves muscle strength

and boosts endurance. Exercise delivers oxygen and nutrients to bodily tissues and supports the cardiovascular system to work more efficiently. And when heart and lung health improve, you have more energy to tackle the daily routine and work. Regular physical activity produces endorphins—chemicals in the brain that improve the ability to sleep, reduce stress and anxiety. For some who suffer from stress on a regular basis, it is crucial to have a way to relax mentally even if it's just a few hours a week.

With today's sedentary lifestyle, particularly where physical activity is lacking, physical tiredness is not experienced, so sleep quality tends to be affected. The advice for a good night's sleep, is to take up a physical activity or work out. The muscles will work to pump some fresh oxygenated blood throughout the veins and brain, and you will experience some tiredness at the end of the workout. The benefits are similar to dance.

<u>Dancing</u> is a very good exercise and a fun activity. This activity really helps to boost the feel good hormones as well as support the maintenance of good bone and muscle mass. It is a good way to maintain a healthy weight and a good mood. It has been proven that learning new dancing skills and other physical activities such as yoga combinations improves memory and enhances concentration, which is beneficial for all ages. According to the recent studies, frequent dancing is a beneficial activity that can help protect against dementia and Alzheimer's disease. It can improve the overall quality of life. Dance exercises combined with healthy nutrition assist weight loss, boost metabolism and help people to stay in shape. Find a style of dance which makes you happy and you actually want to practice even if it's not as energy intensive as you had hoped it would be.

Dance will make you more flexible and graceful in your everyday life. It can also help you become more aware of your body, the way you move, your sense of balance, spacial orientation and boost confidence and self esteem. Those who struggle with balance or sometimes feel awkward in movements and handing things may find dancing very helpful. From a social perspective it is a good way to meet new people and prevent loneliness.

Dancing is useful to tone up the muscles, improve posture and blood flow, which in turn boosts the immune system and overall health. It is very difficult to have a great posture in this day and age with all the mobile phone and computer usage daily. However dance and related social events of any kind make you more aware about how you hold your back, you head, shoulders and so on as good posture will align your bones and joints and it will indeed improve the blood flow to your head and other important areas of your body properly oxygenating internal organs and making you healthier.

Attending to physical activity, work out or dance regularly can make you feel good about yourself and make you more disciplined, fulfilled, confident, and in control of your daily life. Actually, feeling confident and empowered should be a "default setting" for all. It disconnects you from all your problems, giving you the chance to unwind and recover from the stresses of daily life. It's very powerful and its effects on the mind somewhat resembles the effects of feel good hormones as well as forcing you to live in the present. As result of these activities, and physical interactions with other happy people is very beneficial as it improves your mood and increases your overall happiness. In fact, these are some of most important benefits of regularly being active. When you are happy- you feel good. When you feel good - everything around you looks and feels better and it makes you feel even happier. This encourages a better quality of life. Music also has a direct influence on mood. If you want to feel better – start listening to music you enjoy regularly. Upbeat and positive attitude is guaranteed. With today's hectic lifestyles it is essential in life to fit in and make time for fun activities.

<u>Dandelion</u> is another useful herb for detoxification. It's specifically helpful for stimulating the liver, helping it to remove waste and toxins from the blood. This in turn can help with digestion and skin health, since both are connected to the liver. The root has a strong action on the liver and is most typically used for detoxification of the body. The leaves however are mildly diuretic and can help the kidneys to flush out waste. Both contain nutrients that will replenish the body.

<u>Detoxification of the body</u> – This is achieved by allowing longer periods between meals and by avoiding unhealthy snacking and junk foods so the body is supported to maintain a healthy digestive system as well as rid itself of unhealthy undigested food waste and toxins it may be carrying; it is especially beneficial to leave at least

eight hours, between evening meal and breakfast to support the detoxification process. Glutathione is a major detoxifier which the body relies on for clearing toxins. It is produced in the liver. MSM, is an anti-oxidant and an aid in the production of glutathione. This is really a crucial component of MSM as its effectiveness is its ability to increase the production of this important anti-oxidant. N acetyl cystene (NAC) is considered a very efficient supplement owing to its ability to also enhance the production glutathione. Recent studies show that the compounds in stinging nettle can increase glutathione levels, while also protecting the liver from toxins and inflammation. Detoxification and liver health happen to be essential for overall hormone balance and are supported by this effective anti-oxidant. Try to avoid toiletries and products that use chemical ingredients because they are being absorbed and toxify the body. The more natural and the fewer ingredients they have the better.

<u>Diet</u> – A plant based diet rich in fresh fruit and vegetables is very beneficial for health and wellbeing. Try and eat seasonal fruit and vegetables as the seasonal produce provides many health benefits to the body, and there are also benefits to the planet. Try and moderate junk food, frozen and fried foods. If possible try to avoid drinks, foods, skin products and devices which may be harmful for the body: Alcohol, fizzy water and drinks, white refined sugar and sweets, crisps, fried food, trans fats, processed food, table salt and white refined grains such as rice, pasta, bread, pastries. When purchasing food products always check their ingredients in case they may contain harmful substances such as sugar (white refined) or anything that ends with an -ose such as glucose, fructose, sucrose, maltose, harmful sweeteners, food additives, including those that end with -ates or -ites such as in nitrates and nitrites, which are found in processed meats, food colouring, preservatives and any other type of harmful chemical compounds or other compounds such as Tyramine, commonly found in alcoholic beverages, aged cheeses, and meats. Also, if a food product is not certified organic or certified non-GMO and has more than five ingredients listed on the label, odds are high that it does, in fact, contain GMOs. Food products are primarily made up of the first four or five ingredients listed on the label and they are in order of quantity.

<u>Digestive aid tea</u> – A mix of coriander, cumin and fennel seeds. Add one third of a teaspoon of each seed per person. This is extremely

beneficial after meals as an aid to digestion. Lemon, lime and ginger and natural sweetener may also be added to this tea.

<u>Disease prevention</u> is very important. An essential way to achieve this is to eat healthy nourishing foods, reduce the intake of processed, modified, and stale foods. Do not snack in between meals, thus allowing food to digest properly by allowing 4-5 hours between meals, this aids the body to effectively remove toxins, and the undigested food waste build up; which can reverse and prevent disease. Avoid certain food combinations that obstruct metabolic processes, i.e. eat fruit on its own do not mix with other foods as it can lead to food not digesting properly; instead causing a build-up of toxic overload and fat build up. Try and eat seasonal produce as there are benefits to the body and also the planet. Consume cooked foods within an hour of cooking. As leftover food causes stagnation, the system becomes slow and sluggish, this in turn can adversely impact the bodily functions. As well as diet, for disease prevention, it is crucial to regularly detoxify the body and mind. Massage assists with the removal of toxins, environmental pollutants and other accumulated toxins. Other important means for detoxification include the use of ayurvedic or TCM therapies and herbs. As all the systems of the body require cleansing and removal of toxin build up; the blood, liver, lymphatic system, kidneys, digestive and respiratory systems and bowels etc. Herbs such as Nettles address the cleansing function of the adrenals, blood, kidneys and liver, Red clover is used to cleanse toxins away from the blood, lymphatic and respiratory systems. Many herbs have multi-use such as the ones in triphala and are also recommended. The herbs suggested are dependent upon which healing modality is in use and some of these herbs with their uses are discussed in depth.

<u>Dulse</u> – The important health benefits of dulse include its ability to build bone health, optimize the digestive system, increase growth and repair, lower blood pressure, improve vision, and protect the immune system. Dulse is extremely beneficial to rid the body of heavy metal toxins.

<u>Electrolytes</u> are chemicals that regulate nerve and muscle function. Electrolytes hydrate the body, balance blood acidity, blood pressure and help rebuild damaged tissue. These chemicals conduct electricity when mixed with water. The muscles and neurons are referred to

as the "electric tissues" of the body. Important electrolyte minerals are sodium, chloride, potassium, calcium, magnesium, phosphate and bicarbonate. Medication, sickness and diarrhea cause a loss of important electrolytes. It is essential that they are replaced in order for them to continue the important functions mentioned. Electrolytes can be replaced by taking sea or himalayan salts, celery juice, coconut water and lemons amongst others foods.

EMF – Electromagnetic fields arise whenever electricity is used and impact negatively on the physical body. Certain products are available that work to neutralise these fields in the home such as shields, phone magnets, laptop pads etc. Walking on grass barefoot is also extremely beneficial. This practice is used to ground and rebalance the body's magnetic field especially with today's hectic lifestyle with electrical, emf, radio waves everywhere. Also, try to avoid using devices such as microwaves, because the use of this oven may damage the nutrients in food and it may also make some foods toxic. Switch the Wi-Fi off when it is not in use, such as during night-time and sleep as it may damage good microbes, dna and affect overall health. It may also influence the body's natural electric field. An energy field, or electric field, is a physics term used to describe the magnetic fields created in the space surrounding electrically charged particles. Because of the body's electrically charged particles, our cells and tissues generate electrical fields.

The Endocrine system – is referred to as the hormonal system, this is found in many other types of living organisms. This is made up of:

- Glands situated throughout the body;

- Hormones made by the glands and released into the bloodstream or the fluid surrounding cells; and

- Receptors in various organs and tissues that recognize and respond to the hormones.

Ashwagandha and some of the other herbs discussed act as hormonal modulators and act on the endocrine system, encouraging hormonal balance.

Energy – Blackstrap molasses are known to boost energy levels naturally due to their nutritionally dense composition.

Nettles also provide a natural boost for energy due to their iron and amino acid content.

- The body utilizes iron and amino acids to make hemoglobin, (this protein transports oxygen throughout the body);

- By ensuring adequate hemoglobin levels in the body (low when anemic) , the body receives more oxygen;

- More oxygen leads to more energy;

- Additionally, the body uses amino acids to produce energy;

- If essential amino acids are lacking in the diet, more fatigue is experienced;

- Taking stinging nettle supports to naturally increase energy levels, without having to rely on strong stimulants.

<u>Epidermis</u> – The epidermis is the top layer of your skin, Eat healthy fats to keep these tissues healthy.

<u>Epsom Salt Baths</u> – These salts are very beneficial for body and muscular aches and arthritis. The body absorbs the right amount of magnesium. Epsom bath salts are very good for treating stress, promoting relaxation, help with digestion, improve nerve function and aid circulation.

<u>Eucalyptus oil</u> - This oil comes from the eucalyptus tree. It is used as an antiseptic, a perfume, in cosmetics, as a flavoring and is used in dental preparations. Traditional Ayurvedic, Chinese, and Greek, medicines have utilised it in the treatment of a range of conditions for thousands of years as from ancient times it is believed Eucalyptus has a number of medicinal properties, although not all of them have been confirmed by research. Some of its potential health benefits are outlined:

- Eucalyptus oil may stimulate an immune system response; researchers found that Eucalyptus oil specifically; could enhance the immune system's phagocytic cell response to pathogens in a test model. Phagocytosis is a process where the immune system consumes and destroys foreign particles.

- Researchers found evidence supporting the antimicrobial action of eucalyptus. They concluded that that eucalyptus oil may have anti-bacterial effects on pathogenic bacteria in the upper respiratory tract, including Haemophilus influenzae, a bacterium responsible for a range of infections, and some strains of streptococcus. These studies may hopefully and eventually reduce the need for antibiotics.

- The anti-bacterial and antimicrobial potential of eucalyptus has been harnessed for use in some mouthwash and dental preparations. In promoting dental health, eucalyptus appears to be active in fighting bacteria that cause tooth decay and periodontitis.

- Traditional Aboriginal medicines used eucalyptus to treat fungal infections and skin wounds.

- It is a popular home remedy for colds and bronchitis. It may act as an expectorant for loosening phlegm and easing congestion. A number of cough medications include eucalyptus oil. Fresh eucalyptus leaves used in a gargle may be used to relieve a sore throat, sinusitis, and bronchitis. Also, eucalyptus oil vapor appears to act as a decongestant when inhaled.

- Eucalyptus extract may act as a pain reliever, and research indicates that the oil may have analgesic properties. Eucalyptamint, a medicinal preparation, is used to treat muscle and joint pain linked to strains and sprains, arthritis, bruising, and backache.

- Eucalyptus is an effective insect repellent and insecticide. Eucalyptus oil is used as an insecticide and a miticide for killing mites and ticks. Oil of lemon eucalyptus is recommended by some as an insect repellant; it is effective at keeping mosquitoes away. Researchers in India found that eucalyptus oil was active against the larvae and pupae of the housefly and suggested that it could be a viable option for use in eco-friendly products to control houseflies.

- The leaves also contain flavonoids and tannins; flavonoids are plant-based anti-oxidants, and tannins may help to reduce inflammation.

- Other conditions that eucalyptus may assist with include: Arthritis — potentially due to its anti-inflammatory properties: blocked nose and sinus; wounds and burns; ulcers; cold sores — perhaps due to its anti-inflammatory properties; bladder diseases; diabetes — eucalyptus might help lower blood sugar; fever and flu.

<u>Eyes</u> — Keep eyes clean and hydrated every day. Eyesight can be improved with regular eye exercises. An eye bath with triphala can be beneficial for all eye related issues; boil cool and strain the liquid of the herbs thoroughly before using. The recommendation is usually to do this for a month; consult an ayurvedic practitioner. Cupping the eyes with warmed hands for twenty minutes daily as well is beneficial for eye health. There is an acupressure point on the hands between the middle and forefinger to release energy blockages that may help eye health. Ayurvedic practitioners use an eye bath of pure ghee to nourish the eyes, and benefit dry eyes and reduce the red veins in the eyes. Eyebright is useful in the treatment of many eye conditions.

<u>Eye vitamins</u> — Vitamin A, B2, B6, B9, E and Zinc are very beneficial. Omega 3 and Lutein, are valuable nutrients utilised by the body to improve eyesight. Green aventurine is beneficial for eye muscles and can help short sightedness.

<u>Fat</u> — To reduce fat eat less junk food and reduce snacking, as food that is not digested properly can clog the bodily tissues and organs and store an excess of adipose fat.

<u>Fasting</u> — Try not to fast as the body starts to break down muscles once the fat stores have been depleted. Instead eat light nourishing foods for a few days to allow the body to rest and release toxin overload. Allow longer periods between meals if bloating occurs. Eating kitchari twice a week; works as a natural body cleanse and is usually eaten as a replacement to harsh fasting in ayurvedic medicine. As well as nourishing the body, kitchari supports the body with the release of toxins, undigested food waste and pathogens.

<u>Fear / negative emotions</u> — Experience the emotion when it comes up. Try and be present to the emotion, it may happen many times, but

each time you experience it fully, it will go. Try and see the positive aspects of any situation. Fear is usually behind any change; fear will fall away when replaced with gratitude. Replace negative emotions with positive ones by thinking of an event or memory that brings a sense of peace and joy.

Fennel – The cleansing properties of these seeds help in maintaining a healthy gall bladder and liver. Fennel seed tea is beneficial for liver health. These seeds are used to relieve gout, break down kidney stones and uric acid in the tissues. Fennel seed is known as the best medicine for its ability to improve digestion. It is used to treat digestive discomfort, flatulence, cramps, nausea and slow or dull digestion and to alleviate coughs. Fennel bulb is great for cooling down excess heat in the body.

Fenugreek is a spice used for cooking that also has some health benefits to offer. Commonly used in complementary and alternative medicine, fenugreek seed can be taken in supplement form or used to make extracts. The dried seed can also be brewed to make medicinal tea.

As an herbal medicine, fenugreek is believed to prevent or treat a wide range of health conditions, like diabetes, menstrual cramps, an enlarged prostate, and obesity. Fenugreek has also been used for centuries as a substance that can stimulate the production of breast milk (a galactagogue).

Fenugreek seeds and tea are sometimes used to prevent or treat menstrual cramps.

It may also help prevent people with pre-diabetes from progressing to diabetes as some studies suggest that fenugreek seeds may improve blood sugar (glucose) control in people with diabetes.

Fenugreek is a popular folk remedy for stimulating breast milk production. Certain substances in fenugreek are thought to have a similar action to the female hormone estrogen.

It has been suggested that Fenugreek could improve the sex drive (libido) of older males with lower testosterone levels as it contains compounds called furostanolic saponins that may help stimulate the production of the male hormone testosterone.

Some of the health benefits of fenugreek include:

- Reduce the risk of diabetes

- Improve milk production and flow

- Raise testosterone and boost sperm count

- Reduce inflammation

- Pain relief

- Improve weight loss

- Reduce the risk of heart and blood pressure conditions.

<u>Gas</u> – Peppermint assists the body with elimination of gas, but too much of this herb may reduce iron absorption. Chamomile/ginger teas are also beneficial for the body to reduce gas. Triphala when taken regularly is also beneficial for gas reduction.

<u>Ginger</u> – This root is taken to ease the symptoms of osteoarthritis, nausea, cold and flu as well as an upset stomach. Ginger has been used for its medicinal qualities for centuries. Ginger is an anti-inflammatory and is alkaline in ph; this spice ground is used with bicarbonate of soda in the bath to ease aching muscles as well as help with circulation and acidity problems. Ginger is generally a warming root, drank in tea with lemon aids digestion.

<u>Glucosamine</u> is a compound that is naturally produced by the body. It is found in plant foods. The vegan supplements are plant or corn derived. Most commonly, it exists in the cartilage and assists to create the proteins and fats that repair cartilage when it is damaged.

Glucosamine is not commonly found in foods, but it is often sold as a supplement in drops, capsules, or topical forms. Taking vegan glucosamine supplements may offer health benefits, particularly for joint pain such as arthritis. Glucosamine supplements can provide some important health benefits. Early trials suggest that glucosamine may have some anti-oxidant effects that can improve eye health, which is especially useful for people with conditions like glaucoma.

Furthermore, glucosamine can provide benefits like: reduced joint pain, particularly among people with osteoarthritis. Supplements of combined glucosamine and phytodroitin — (a related compound also found in cartilage as chondroitin), — have been shown to be as effective as osteoarthritis treatments. As certain people do not react well to non-steroidal anti-inflammatory drugs, glucosamine supplements may be a safe and effective way to reduce symptoms of arthritis. Vegan glucosamine and phytodroitin supplements may also help reduce chronic inflammation, which is linked to a number of potential health problems like arthritis, diabetes as well as heart disease. This may be part of the reason why glucosamine reduces arthritis pain. Studies have linked regular consumption of glucosamine supplements with lower levels of inflammation. Regularly taking the supplements can help lower your risk of a number of chronic conditions. With current research, early studies suggest that glucosamine supplements may assist with the prevention and the progression of osteoporosis post-menopause. Essentially, glucosamine seems to reduce the weakening of bones by supporting healthy bone growth. This makes the supplements especially helpful for people who are at risk of developing osteoporosis as they age.

Glucosamine has shown to possess some skin benefits such as: treat hyperpigmentation, wound healing, wrinkle reduction, and it may provide moisture for the skin.

<u>Goji Berries</u> – The Chinese have used goji berries for over 6000 years to boost the immune system, protect the eyes and to protect against free radicals and ageing. Goji Berries contain the highest number of amino acids found, and these berries are also the only super food to encourage the pituitary gland to emancipate the human growth hormone (HGH) in the body. Due to the large amounts of vitamin c also present in the berry, taking too much may cause diarrhea.

<u>Golden Milk</u> – Hot milk with ½ tsp turmeric helps to reduce inflammation and also heal internal injury in the body.

<u>Good posture</u> – It is important to ensure good posture for a healthy back and body. A person will feel more confident with the support of a good posture. A healthy posture will reduce the risk of neck, shoulder and back pain with less chance of developing a double chin!

<u>Gout</u> can be relieved by ensuring adequate blood flow to the area in pain. Cherries are beneficial in treating the inflammation of gout.

<u>Grass</u> – Walking on grass barefoot is extremely beneficial as this practice offers to ground and rebalance the body's magnetic field especially with today lifestyle with electrical, emf, radio waves everywhere.

<u>Gratitude</u> – Practicing gratitude is an activation of positivity that encourages you to take the time to express kindness, or share a positive response to the world, other people or an act of generosity. Gratitude encourages you to be appreciative of what you have and recognise that good things exist outside of yourself. But, even without this evidence, acknowledging that you are grateful for something, like sunshine, will help to make you and those around you feel more positive. Although it can time and patience to develop new habits; the same principal applies when learning the habit of gratitude and quietening the mind. We are programmed to constantly desire more material objects, so instead of contentment we experience lack as we're more focused on lack. It may be difficult to be grateful when there are problems in day to day life, such as money, health related issues etc, and life is not always easy; a valuable to way to approach change is to learn a sense of appreciation and to distinguish the positive aspects of each situation.

There are numerous benefits from the daily practice of gratitude; such as contentment; a stronger immune system; better sleep and a sense of well-being and many other benefits.

<u>Graviola</u> – A tree that is native to the Amazon rainforest that produces edible fruits. Its bark, leaf, root and stem are also beneficial due to the high level of anti-oxidants it can assist the body to fight free radical damage and help reduce inflammation. Graviola contains minerals and vitamins B1, B2, magnesium and zinc that support the body to fight bugs and keep ill health away. With its high concentration of vitamins and minerals Graviola is beneficial for bone health. Graviola is able to enhance the immune systems capability in fighting bugs, fungus, virus, bacteria and most known pathogens.

<u>Green tea</u> is a natural source of caffeine. Green tea is packed with healthy anti-oxidants. It is great for weight loss especially the matcha variety and has the potential to reduce inflammation.

<u>Grey hair</u> is hair that lacks pigment. This is usually due to a reduction in catalase, a chemical required in maintaining natural hair colour, over

time this does reduce and hydrogen peroxide may increase resulting in grey hair. However there are ways catalase may be increased using some of the methods previously discussed. A recent study showed quantitive evidence linking stress to greying hair in people. It seems stress may accelerate greying hair and research has found that hair colour may be restored, when stressed is eliminated.

<u>Hair loss</u> – There could be many causes of hair loss that include diet, mineral deficiency, protein malnutrition, medications, stress, pollution, ill health and genetics. Another form of hair loss is Alopecia this condition is produced by the autoimmune destruction of hair follicles in localised areas of the skin. A diagnosis may determine the prognosis. Ayurvedic practitioners may prescribe some of the herbal remedies and treatments as discussed before.

Further information and other ways to reverse hair loss are suggested below.

- Diet and supplements. Eating a balanced diet may support healthy hair and hair regrowth. Treat dietary deficiencies: Low levels of iron, vitamins such as B complex, folic acid, minerals and proteins in the diet and vitamin D deficiency may lead to the weakening of hair. This must be identified and treated on time.

- Biotin, also known as vitamin H, B complex vitamins help the body convert food into energy. Studies have suggested that including biotin-rich food in the diet or taking biotin supplements may slow hair loss. For problems with hair fall, include biotin-rich foods such as bananas, nuts, sweet potatoes, onions, and oats in your diet.

- Avoid colouring hair with harsh chemical dyes and stay hydrated as the hair shaft requires water to produce new hair.

- Physical activity: Regular physical activity such as walking for 30 minutes a day helps balance hormonal levels, reduce stress levels besides reducing hair fall.

- Pumpkin seed oil, may reduce the effects of 5-alpha reductase, which is an enzyme that contributes to hair loss and massages also help circulation and blood flow in the scalp. Other herbal remedies are discussed in detail in earlier sections.

- Stress: Studies in the past have found medical evidence to link stress with hair loss. De-stress yourself; one of the ways is using alternative therapy such as meditation and yoga they not only reduce stress but also restore hormonal balance and reduce hair fall problems.

- Telogen effluvium: This is a temporary condition seen in both men and women. Severe hair loss is seen after a period of extreme emotional stress or illness. This type of hair fall is usually reversible. Telogen phase refers to resting phase.

- Anagen effluvium Hair fall can be defined as when hair growth (anagen phase) is hindered. Certain environmental triggers, illnesses and heavy metal toxins cause this type of hair loss. This can be temporary if treated.

- Thyroid problems: Overactive thyroid gland or hypoactive thyroid gland are both known to cause hair loss. The thyroid conditions must be identified and treated in time.

- Prevent traction alopecia: Certain head wear such as hats and caps are used on a regular basis, certain hairstyles such as ponytails, braids, and artificial hairstyles pull hair or tug hair follicles and can eventually cause localised baldness.

- Reduce alcoholic beverages, avoid smoking and heat styling as the amount of blood that flows to the scalp is reduced, and this causes a reduction in hair growth.

Alopecia – As discussed - Loss of hair from the scalp or any part of the body. The condition, usually, occurs when the immune system destroys the hair follicles that results in hair loss. This can be treated by medical or Ayurvedic practitioners with some of the herbal remedies mentioned before.

Nettle is beneficial for skin and hair, as collagen is a major component of hair and skin; Nettle contains amino acids (the building blocks of collagen), but it is also rich in vitamin C (which stimulates collagen production). Nettle is abundant in various trace minerals that are needed for hair growth and preventing wrinkles. In particular, nettles contain silica which is used for collagen production and is responsible for making hair shiny and resilient.

- The hormone DHT (dihydrotestosterone). DHT is an androgen (male hormone) that contributes to alopecia, as well as baldness in both women and men. And one promising study shows that stinging nettle is able to block the enzyme that makes DHT, thereby improving hair growth.

- High androgens are also a factor in PCOS symptoms, acne and excessive facial hair growth. Lastly nettles contain B-vitamins which work together with collagen to keep hair and skin healthy.

- Nettle tea may be used internally, and as a hair rinse, due to its potential to re-grow hair.

- With their many benefits nettles can help provide some relief when consumed regularly.

Coconut or sesame oil, (with their moisturising and nourishing properties), when used with various other herbal ingredients can address particular hair related issues. The herbs are used to treat:

- Lemon keeps the scalp clean and gets rid of dandruff

- Mehendi (Henna) makes hair soft and smooth

- Amla strengthens the roots of hair

- Hibiscus makes hair black

<u>Heart health</u> – Take regular exercise at least 20 minutes a day. Taking an early morning walk in a natural environment away from pollution is especially beneficial. Cherries are very beneficial for cardiovascular health.

<u>Haematococcus pluvial</u> – This is a seaweed rich in a beta carotene also known as asthaxanthin. Because it contains high levels of anti-oxidants, Asthaxanthin supports the body's functions to balance inflammation, support anti-ageing, minimise age related illness, reduce diabetes, decrease high blood pressure and high cholesterol. This powerful anti-oxidant produces a beneficial

impact on organs and eye health; it supports the body with the maintenance of brain health as it enhances the regeneration of all cells. Studies have shown this product has been able to reduce brain cell damage and increase blood flow to the brain. It may in some affect calcium absorption.

<u>Haritaki</u> – This ayurvedic herb offers plenty of benefits and has been widely used for centuries in ayurvedic medicine in the East. It is known to do wonders for rejuvenation and mental health. It is a useful blood cleanser and a good metabolic aid. The paste of this herb is useful in reducing swelling, cleansing, purifying, and healing wounds and ulcers. Haritaki may assist in the prevention of digestive and urinary diseases, skin problems, diabetes, constipation, colic pain, ulcers, vomiting, hemorrhoids, heart disease, and irregular fevers.

<u>He shou woo</u> – This Chinese herb is useful in the treatment of hair loss and for premature greying hair. He Shou Wu benefits include improved liver, kidney health and is used as an aid for constipation.

<u>Heat in body in excess</u> – Sheetali pranayama is usually practiced to reduce excess heat in the body in the summer time, but is not practiced excessively during the winter months. Peppermint tea and Bhringraj can have a cooling effect on the body.

<u>Honey</u> – There are countless benefits of taking honey. It is usually recommended to use honey that is produced by a local farmer. Honey contains anti-oxidants and some nutrients such as iron, calcium, magnesium, potassium, also some phosphates. It is an anti-microbial, and anti-bacterial. Using honey to replace refined and processed sugars is very beneficial to health.

Honey has many uses; the only exception is not to cook honey as it is best to use in its raw form. It can be taken in warm but not hot water first thing in the morning to promote cleansing of the body.

<u>Humour</u> – Laughter is a powerful emotional therapy which is a good way to de-stress; elevate the mood; boost the immune system and reduce anger. Laughter is a very good way to release worry and pent up emotions. Regularly entertain the activities that make you laugh.

<u>IBS</u> – Aloe vera juice and eating sensibly inevitably combat the symptoms of IBS.

<u>Indigo</u> can be used with a combination of bhringraj and brahmi to colour hair naturally.

<u>Inflammation</u> – Coriander contains properties that reduce inflammation in the body. Tulsi herb and turmeric offer similar benefits to decrease inflammation throughout the body. Inflammation is an indicator of ill health. A reduction in stress levels does have an impact in the reduction of inflammation. Pathogens, viruses, bacteria and mould also contribute to inflammation and some auto-immune disorders. MSM may prove useful in managing inflammation. Commonly its use is most often to try to treat arthritis, as it is usually taken to relieve arthritis pain.

Inflammation is the body's natural way of fighting off stress. Stress could be emotional, physical or dietary (inflammatory foods, refined sugar, gm foods, hydrogenated fats, pesticides, etc). Stress always triggers the inflammatory response; during the inflammatory response, the following events occur in the body, such as:

- The adrenals glands release cortisol;

- There is an increase in the body's blood sugar levels;

- Simultaneously, thyroid function goes down; this is fine in the short-term, but if stress lingers for a long time, the result is chronic inflammation. Chronic inflammation means theses points all become the body's new "normal."So, lowering inflammation is essential to balancing the hormones naturally and nettles can be a great solution because they are anti-inflammatory.

Nettle leaf lowers inflammation in two ways:

- Nettles support the liver, kidneys and adrenal glands; due to its effect on the adrenal glands it reduces stress, further more due to its effect on the liver and kidneys, the body can get rid of toxins. Fewer toxins equal less inflammation.

- Furthermore, research shows that nettle can relieve joint pain and inflammation, including the pain associated with conditions like arthritis.

- Nettles contain compounds that act like insulin and as a result, they improve blood sugar levels. This is a major benefit for hormonal health because symptoms and conditions like systemic inflammation are tied to elevated blood sugar levels.

<u>Joint care</u> – Ensure healthy eating to include foods containing calcium, copper, selenium, zinc, and healthy fats. Exercise especially brisk walking is good for joint care. It is essential to ensure lubrication of joints is maintained. Glucosamine chondroitin is effective in lubricating the joints to decrease inflammation. Plant derived versions of this supplement are effective in offering a significant reduction in positive mediators of inflammation and assist in increasing the production of hyaluronic acid which is a component of synovial fluid. This fluid helps in lubricating the joints to help rebuild cartilage. Glucosamine is found naturally in the human body; it is a crystalline compound that occurs widely in the connective tissue.

<u>Kapalbhati Pranayama</u> – The benefits of this practice include: An increase in metabolic rate and weight loss; due to stimulation of abdominal organs this is especially beneficial for those with diabetes; it supports improved blood circulation and adds radiance to the face; it improves digestive tract functioning, absorption and assimilation of nutrients. This breathing technique results in a taut and trimmed down belly. Other benefits of this practice include an energised nervous system, rejuvenation of brain cells and a calmer and uplifted mind. As with all pranayama practices caution is advised and these practices should be learnt from a suitably qualified practitioner as adverse effects may be experienced with incorrect practice.

<u>Knee pain</u> – The use of maha narayanan oil and kapalbhati pranayama is beneficial for knee pain. Rubbing the knees with sesame oil and salt prior to taking a hot bath may decrease knee pain. A bath with turmeric, or ginger powder and bicarbonate of soda will also ease the pain and inflammation. Cold showers ease pain and inflammatory conditions over time.

<u>Liver</u> – It is important to detoxify the body. Herbs like Bhumyamalaki are used to treat liver inflammation, liver ailments. Bhumyamalaki is especially used as an aid in liver and kidney recovery. This herb has an ability to cleanse, detoxify, and strengthen this essential organ. Eating properly assists the herbs to work efficiently and reduce toxicity. MSM, N-Acetyl cysteine and Nettle all assist liver function and are discussed in depth.

<u>Love ♡ yourself</u> – Talk to yourself as if you are talking to a friend. If you were actually talking to a friend, could you get away with the things you are saying to yourself? Do not criticise yourself or others. Children are scolded or told off for something, and when this happens to a child in many cases it is a big deal and is misinterpreted as I am not loved! So as adults we carry these experiences but only from a negative point of view. It is important to understand if there are any negative memories, try to feel safe and loved in the present! Remind yourself frequently you are more than good enough especially in situations when you may lack confidence.

<u>Maca</u> – As a highly nutritious root powder, Maca can aid in fertility for both men and women. It supports the balance of hormones for menopausal women and boosts energy levels, as well as reducing the effects of stress. Maca is able to boost bone health and improve the skin and the immune system as it contains B vitamins and certain minerals. Long-term use supports a normal balance of hormones; physical and emotional health are also improved.

<u>Magnesium</u> – Magnesium is an extremely important mineral that is required by the body to maintain optimal health. It is one of the most abundant minerals in the body and is absolutely essential for the regulation of hundreds of biochemical reactions. Every cell in the body needs this mineral, especially if you suffer from panic, or have joint and muscle pain or cramps you may be deficient of this mineral. To restore magnesium, probably the easiest way to obtain this mineral is through Epsom bath salts, as these salts are rich in magnesium. This mineral is also obtained by including avocado, legumes and tofu in the diet. Magnesium is necessary for healthy muscles including the heart, muscles and bones as it ensures calcium absorption. This mineral may prevent migraines and constipation. Other benefits include prevention of asthma, a decrease in high blood pressure and insomnia and sleep issues are resolved.

<u>Meditation</u> – Many benefits are derived from regular meditation practice for mental and physical health as well as neurological health benefits. Meditation balances both hemispheres of the brain; it assists with the regulation of the specialised brain centers that control emotions such as anxiety, fear, panic and bodily sensations of hunger and pain. This practice can help manage anxiety, reduce stress, reduce depression and promote emotional health. With

regular meditation many other beneficial habits can develop; feelings such as a positive mood and outlook in life, healthy sleep patterns, self discipline, strength and an increased tolerance of pain.

Meditation is now used as a scientific solution to treat modern lifestyle stressors as it can create happiness and a sense of well-being within a person. This practice improves the cognitive abilities of individuals, it improves self esteem, self image and self worth and it offers a heightened attention and concentration span. Meditation improves health by controlling the alpha brain waves. The alpha waves in the brain operate the way we use our sense organs and respond to external stimulations.

Taking into consideration the many distractions we have, meditation helps sharpen focus and concentration. Meditation stimulates the brain centers to produce more of the feel good hormones and build an immunity to modern diseases. Meditation is extremely beneficial for ADHD as it offers numerous benefits and assists focus and concentration and reduces hyperactivity. The beneficial effects of long-term meditation are cumulative. In order to obtain the full benefits of meditation it is essential to learn this practice from a suitably qualified complete teacher.

- Meditation improves physical health by boosting the immune functions, regulating hormonal discharge, and decreasing cellular inflammation.

- Some research has found that the effects of long-term meditation can produce more disease-fighting chemicals in the body than no-meditation.

- Some fertility studies showed that women who meditated were more fertile and delivered healthier babies than women who did not.

- Nervous breakdowns and panic attacks can be prevented by using meditation. As meditation regulates the sympathetic and autonomic nervous systems and so meditation controls our responses during sudden stress encounters.

- Meditation stabilizes blood circulation in the body and regulates blood pressure, heartbeat, metabolism, and other essential biological functioning.

- By bringing a positive shift in lifestyle, meditation improves sleep quality, helps weight loss, and reduces fatigue.

<u>Mental health</u> – Ashwagandha is known as an aid for depression. It alleviates problems associated with memory impairment by protecting the brain against oxidative stress. Regular pranayama practice, exercise and meditation also provide benefits to alleviate mental health and depression. Therapies such as NLP and Cognitive behavioral therapy may help with chronic mental health issues.

<u>Menthol</u> may be used as an anti-inflammatory; as it works as an analgesic for the relief of pain for arthritis symptoms. Menthol is mainly used as a decongestant for colds, throat, chest and flu.

<u>Metabolism</u> – Metabolism is the set of life-sustaining chemical reactions in organisms. The three main purposes of metabolism are: the conversion of the energy in food to energy available to run cellular processes; the conversion of food to building blocks for proteins, and some carbohydrates; and the elimination of metabolic waste.

<u>Mindfulness</u> – It is important to try and remain in the present moment; this can help ease stress and worry.

Practicing mindfulness can bring improvements in both physical and psychological symptoms as well as positive changes in health, attitudes, and behaviors.

- Benefits of mindfulness on mental health. In recent years, psychotherapists have turned to mindfulness meditation as an important technique as a treatment of a number of problems, including: depression, substance abuse, eating disorders, couples' conflicts, anxiety disorders, and OCD (obsessive-compulsive disorder) as well as improve mood and over thinking.

- Mindfulness affects on physical health: Scientists have discovered that mindfulness techniques assist to improve physical health in a number of ways. Mindfulness can: relieve stress, treat heart disease, lower blood pressure, reduce chronic pain, improve sleep, and alleviate gastrointestinal difficulties.

- Mindfulness for wellbeing - Increasing your capacity for mindfulness supports many attitudes these contribute to a satisfied life. Being mindful, encourages you become fully engaged in activities, and creates a greater capacity to deal with adverse events. By focusing on the here and now, many people who practice mindfulness find that they are less likely to get caught up in worries about the future or regrets over the past, are less preoccupied with concerns about success and self-esteem, and are better able to form deep connections with others.

Mint – There are different varieties of mint the most popular ones are Peppermint and Spearmint. These herbs have been in use since ancient times, due to their medicinal properties. Peppermint and Spearmint are still regularly used in most cultures and have different properties.

Peppermint (*Mentha x Piperitais*) is a type of hybrid mint, reproduced through a combination of spearmint and watermint. It has a spicy refreshing flavor that makes it a popular ingredient in many different foods, toothpaste and sweets among others. The leaves of this plant are the main parts that are used, due to the presence of the essential oil, which contains high levels of menthone, menthol, limonene, and various other acids, compounds, and anti-oxidants. Due to these properties peppermint improves colds and flu, headaches, indigestion, IBS, nausea, skin conditions and vomiting during pregnancy.

Spearmint – The properties of this herb include a combination of anti-bacterial, anti-oxidant, phytocompounds and carvone compounds. The phytocompounds within the spearmint plant are thought to support digestive health. Due to the compound carvone spearmint can help limit muscle contractions in the digestive tract, which can help relieve indigestion and support healthy digestive function.

Plant compounds within spearmint enable the body's endocrine system to balance hormone production. The endocrine system uses hormones to send signals throughout the body. This system plays an essential role in regulating body function. Chemical compounds in spearmint can work with our own chemical hormones to help maintain balance within. Evidence suggests that after drinking spearmint tea twice a day for a month, the herb's compounds may reduce testosterone while increasing ovulation-related hormones such as luteinizing hormone, follicle-stimulating hormone and estradiol and provide hormonal regulation support for women.

It may support cognitive function as studies have shown the regular use of Spearmint supports an increase in alertness, focus and memory. Other benefits of spearmint includes: aids digestion; assist women with hormone balancing; normalise blood sugar; aids respiratory health; aids circulation; heart health and stress and tension relief.

<u>Moods</u> – To elevate the mood maintain a healthy balance by engaging with others, exercising, smiling and eating the right food.

<u>Moringa</u> is known as the miracle tree. There are many benefits of Moringa use as it contains many nutrients. It protects the skin and nourishes the hair. Moringa is a good stabiliser of mood and has a positive effect on heart and neurotransmitter activity. Other benefits of taking Moringa regularly include a reduction of tiredness and fatigue.

<u>MSM</u>, also known as methylsulfonylmethane. Organic MSM is found in fresh raw foods. Plant foods high in MSM include Brussels sprouts, garlic, onions, asparagus, legumes, kale and wheat germ. Then continue with Vegan MSM – the compound used in supplements – is a highly concentrated white, crystalline powder and contains 34% sulphur. This is a mineral which we are largely deficient in due to the poor mineral concentrations in the majority of soils today. Even if you eat large quantities of plants high in sulfur, it's still likely you may be deficient in this super-food. Benefits of Vegan MSM include:

- MSM is a natural analgesic (pain reliever) and an anti-inflammatory. It also increases cellular permeability and dilates blood vessels, increasing circulation and the removal of waste products from the cells, decreasing time needed to heal from injury and wounds. MSM is also a muscle relaxant.

- MSM aids in the absorption of vitamin C, all B vitamins, CoQ10, amino acids, calcium, magnesium, and more and so works as a synergist.

- A result of its anti-oxidant abilities, particularly sulfur, MSM, acts as an aid in the production of glutathione – one of the key anti-oxidants in reducing oxidative stress.

- Due to this compounds detoxification abilities it aids in the removal of heavy metal toxicity and cellular waste products. In addition, the production of glutathione assists the liver in removing waste products from the body.

- This compound can extend the blood-brain barrier, as it improves neurological function, so improving cellular function and removing heavy metal toxicity within the brain cells which may also improve memory.

- MSM reduces and relieves allergies, due to its work as an antihistamine and works to heal the mucosa within the gastrointestinal and urogenital tracts as well as the respiratory system. This decreases the availability for allergen, pathogen, and parasite binding.

- It reduces the severity of auto-immune disorders due to its analgesic, anti-inflammatory, detoxification, mucosal healing, and anti-oxidant effects. MSM helps to decrease auto-immune reactions, particularly in and around joints and connective tissue.

- It helps to balance blood sugar, the sulfur is needed for proper structure and function of insulin, essential in carbohydrate metabolism.

- MSM reduces muscle soreness and cramps when taken prior to training. When consumed after training, MSM aids in reducing muscle cramps and increasing recovery between training sessions. MSM may reduce post-training muscle soreness and delayed onset muscle soreness.

- It also beautifies skin, hair, and nails as sulfur is needed in the production of collagen and keratin — two proteins required for healthy hair, skin, and nails. It keeps the skin smooth, soft and youthful looking and the hair shiny as well as assisting with the reduction of hair-loss and alopecia.

<u>Neem</u> – Due to the beneficial anti-bacterial, anti-fungal and anti-viral qualities of neem, it helps to get rid of infections, intestinal worms, protects skin, teeth and gums. It is a common pest repellent and can slow down the ageing process. Neem is also very beneficial to clear acne and pimples.

<u>N-acetylcysteine</u> (NAC), is an amino acid naturally produced in the body. NAC is naturally found in legumes. It may reduce inflammation and is effective for detoxification of the body. Taking it as a supplement may help improve symptoms of a number of medical conditions.

- It is considered a very effective supplement in vegan form owing to its ability to enhance the production of one of the body's most effective anti-oxidants; an enzyme called glutathione. This is really highlights its effectiveness; due to its ability to increase production of this important anti-oxidant, NAC has the ability to protect against cell decay and the resultant complications and diseases. It can also play a vital role in boosting the body's immune system and there have been a variety of studies demonstrating that a reduced glutathione level is linked to immune system disorders. It should be taken an hour or so after other vitamins and supplements as it may affect their absorption.

- NAC has long been used to help dissolve mucus in those suffering from chronic respiratory complaints. It has also been administered with great success by protecting the liver from the toxins. This important anti-oxidant helps protect the body's cellular integrity and assists to repair damage done by the free radicals that are encountered on a daily basis. Free radical damage is considered to be one of the major factors contributing towards heart disease, terminal illness and other degenerative diseases.

- This amino acid may protect against many of the signs of aging because of its potent anti-oxidant abilities including macular degeneration and cataracts both of which are heavily linked to oxidative stress. NAC supplementation may help boost anti-oxidant activities in both the macula and the lens of the eye protecting them against free radical damage that cause cataracts.

- NAC supplements can help treat and ease a variety of respiratory conditions including asthma, bronchitis and sinusitis. NAC has been used for a number of years by allopathic doctors to dilute the consistency of mucus in order to help patients eliminate it with ease either by coughing or draining. It has proven especially useful in treating bad congestion in people suffering from chronic respiratory complaints such as pneumonia. NAC has demonstrated the ability to lessen the severity of flu and its duration.

- Experts suggest NAC may have a role to play on prevention of terminal illness because of its anti-oxidant ability to fight the cellular damage caused by free radicals and its ability to eliminate environmental toxins. A study has concluded that NAC supplements may reduce the adverse effects of the treatments involved in treating these illnesses. Evidence suggests it can reduce the levels of certain compounds such as homocysteine which are linked to cardiac diseases. Being a potent anti-oxidant, NAC may also prevent oxidation and prevent the build-up of LDL or the bad cholesterol so it is beneficial for heart health.

- NAC generally assists to protect the body against environmental toxins and promotes their removal via the liver due to providing assistance with producing the anti-oxidant, glutathione. A few toxic substances that NAC can help combat include alcohol, chloroform, chromium, carbon monoxide, and mercury.

- This amino acid seems to be a viable option for chronic conditions in the liver. Various medications have been tried in the treatment of these acute viral conditions, a few studies have concluded positive outcomes from patients taking NAC, for these conditions. More recently, studies have shown positive results with the absence of side effects in patients treated with NAC.

High doses of NAC may present side effects such as it may contribute to fever, gastrointestinal disorders, vomiting or a reduction to the glutathione actually being produced in the body. Those taking blood thinning medications should avoid NAC as it may cause blood clotting issues.

<u>Nettle Tea</u> – Stinging nettle is a weed that grows worldwide, during contact fresh nettle leaves release a chemical that stings; once the

herb is dried the stinging effect is removed. Ayurvedic medicine use nettle as a nourishing and rejuvenative tonic particularly for kidneys and adrenals, it increases vitality. By stimulating the liver and kidneys, nettle assists to clear toxins from undigested food waste, and tightens and strengthens the blood vessels, purifies the blood and assists healthy heart function. Nettle is known as a super food with many benefits to offer. As a rich source of iron, it has traditionally been used in the treatment of anemia and is an excellent source of: Vitamins A, C and K. It is also a source of Fatty acids, and also minerals like iron, calcium, potassium, manganese and proteins. In addition, nettles are high in chlorophyll. Chlorophyll is great for detoxification. Furthermore, stinging nettle is loaded with anti-oxidants including carotenoids, flavonoids and phenolic compounds, such as: Beta carotene, Lutein, Quercetin, Rutin and B Vitamins, vitamin E, protein and many more nutrients.

Nettles assist the detoxification process and reduce systemic inflammation. By reducing excess heat in the body they can assist inflammatory skin conditions like acne, rosacea and eczema.

<u>Nutritional Yeast</u> is a very beneficial source of vitamins and minerals; it contains all nine essential amino acids making it a complete protein and it is low in saturated fat. Complete proteins are important as they assist functions such as tissue repair, nutrient absorption and prevention of muscle loss. This yeast combats brittle nails and hair loss. Taking this yeast regularly improves skin conditions and reduces acne. This yeast is a great source of source of b vitamins and vitamin b12.

<u>Oiling of belly button</u> aims to release the knots and tangles in the belly button. This is done by applying various oils to the belly button. There are benefits of oiling the belly button, as there are 72000 nerves all behind the belly button that correspond to the rest of the body and its organs. An imbalance is usually detected by the appearance, size, and shape of the belly button. Oiling is used to assist many different ailments from e.g. ghee for dry eyes, almond oil for glowing skin, rose water to enhance skin tone and to regenerate skin cells, honey for dry skin, lemon oil for clear skin, castor oil for knee pain. Various different oils are used the oils offer different benefits depending on the ailment.

<u>Oil pulling</u> – An ancient Indian medicinal remedy, the process involves swishing oil around the month 10-20 minutes using sesame or

coconut oil. It can improve oral health, tooth decay, bleeding gums and general health by removing unhealthy bacteria and toxins. Some say it has helped with headaches and migraine, diabetes, asthma, jaw health and other ailments. Oil pulling has been used successfully for thousands of years, as modern sugars and grains have been shown to weaken tooth enamel.

<u>Olive Leaf</u> is a staple of the Mediterranean diet. Scientists study this extract for its potential to prevent chronic diseases. Research points to lower rates of illnesses. It is a potent source of anti-oxidants that support the immune system. Olive leaf extract is a concentrated dose of all the nutrients in olive tree leaves.

By fighting cell damage that causes disease, anti-oxidants work to reduce the risks of many illnesses. The anti-oxidants in olive leaf extract are mainly polyphenols. These plant-based nutrients play a role in preventing conditions such as cognitive decline, Olive leaf also contains a uniquely powerful polyphenol called <u>oleuropein</u>. Studies show that in addition to its anti-oxidant activity, oleuropein has anti-inflammatory, anti-viral, and anti-microbial effects. These properties point to research backed health benefits such as: Improved cardiovascular health, lower risk of diabetes and a stronger immune system. Olive leaf extract supports this function thanks to oleuropein's ability to attack and neutralise viruses and bacteria.

<u>Oranges</u> are very good for eyesight if you eat one a day. Oranges are rich in vitamin A and Vitamin C which is good for heart health and it helps to bolster the immune system.

<u>Oregano oil</u> – Do not use oregano essential oil as it should not be taken internally only pure oregano oil should be consumed. This oil is useful as an anti-bacterial, anti-viral and anti-fungus. Take 2-4 drops in a glass of water, do not exceed use for more than three days at a time as oregano oil may affect gut health. Have a break and then continue use if required for a further three days. Oregano oil may be taken as an anti-viral; it works as a natural antibiotic and symptoms usually start to decrease within a few days. Be sure to top up with good probiotic to ensure a healthy gut with plenty of beneficial gut bacteria.

<u>Over thinking</u> – It is useful to empty the mind of all thoughts regularly in order to focus on the present and think logically.

<u>Panchkarma</u> is considered as the classic Ayurvedic detoxification treatment and it involves five independent cleansing processes simultaneously to ensure a radical detoxification. The aim of these treatments is to ensure that the body's vital energies can flow freely again. At the same time, the constitutions of the body are also restored to their natural equilibrium. This practice enhances the patient's sense of well-being as it also helps the body's own defences to combat lots of different illnesses. Many people choose to undergo a regular Ayurvedic detoxification therapy. The panchakarma program consists of five cleansing and healing therapies that help restore balance and strengthen the immune system and is specific to the individual's constitution.

- Basti, which uses herbal enemas to purge the large intestines;

- Raktamokshana, purifies the blood;

- Nasya, which is the method used to clean the nasal passage;

- Vamana, removes toxins in the stomach;

- Virechana, removes toxins from the small intestines;

<u>Pranayama positivity</u> – Learn these breathing techniques from a trained authority. These breathing techniques provide immense benefits to general health.

<u>Probiotics</u> are micro-organisms made up of bacteria and fungus, sometimes known as the friendly flora. There are at least 500 different strains of bacteria and fungus in the body. The intestines house up to about 4 pounds of micro-organisms. When this friendly flora lives in harmony in the body it benefits us in many ways:

Science backed research suggests that gut health is the foundation for good health. Nourishment of these bacteria in the gut is important as they are linked with every organ in the body in relation to good health and well-being.

- These live micro-organisms all act on different areas of health in many ways, such as hormonal health which is also linked to gut health. A natural way of obtaining these healthy gut bacteria is through diet by regularly consuming fermented foods, kimchi, plant based foods, yeast, sauerkraut, live yoghurt and having regular contact with dirt. Fat protects the live bacteria to get through acidic environment in the stomach, sugar should be avoided.

- These friendly microbes assist the body by creating a protective lining. This coats the intestines prohibiting "unfriendly microbes" from setting up habitation on the intestinal wall. Most of the energy of the intestinal lining is produced as a result of the bacterial fermentation process. By competing for food, probiotics keep infectious organisms in check.

- Probiotics stimulate the immune system; they produce chemicals that keep harmful microbes away and keep yeast infections such as candida in balance.

- Probiotics ease and prevent constipation and diarrhea and reduce the risk of inflammatory bowel disorder. These microbes assist with the final stage of digestion of fats and proteins.

- Probiotics contain micro-organisms that assist with creating vitamins the body needs like B1, B2, B6, B12, folic acid and biotin.

- This friendly flora detoxifies certain poisons in the digestive tract such as ammonia, cholesterol, excess hormones and other toxins.

Unfortunately there are compounds that can disrupt that balance of gut flora such as: antibiotics, chlorine in water, Birth Control Pills, NSAIDS, ibuprophen, aspirin and many other medicines.

Other pro-biotic disruptors include: Heavily cooked foods; hydrogenated fats and oils, high fructose Corn Syrup, GM produce, refined grains, refined sugars and stress.

Probiotics will benefit, people with food or respiratory allergies, skin problems, yeast issues of any kind, like athlete's foot, thrush infection, nail fungus and dandruff. The micro-organisms can also assist people with a weakened immune system, frequent colds, infections and congestion, as well as anyone with inflammatory bowel disorders and constipation, infants and children to reduce incidence of infection. Especially babies born by c-section as they are unable to pick up any of the mothers flora when passing through the birth canal.

Antibiotics kill off both the bad bacteria and the good bacteria in the body. So it's essential to re-establish the good bacteria with probiotics. Probiotics may be taken during the course of antibiotics. Leave a few hours apart from the antibiotic; otherwise the antibiotics will kill off the good bacteria in the probiotics. They are best taken on an empty stomach rather than with meals as the increased stomach acid necessary to digest food will also kill of the good bacteria in the probiotics. It may be easier to take them while the stomach is empty. If you take them on waking wait at least 20 minutes or so before eating or drinking.

Probiotics are available in fermented or cultured raw foods, such as vinegar, yoghurt, lassi, cultured soy: miso, tempeh fermented beverages such as kombucha, pickled vegetables such as pickles, sauerkraut and sourdough. They can be taken as supplements, usually with multiple strains found in the probiotics. The active cultures can't survive high temperatures.

<u>Qigong</u> – Builds up bone density, slows down the ageing process and improves health. It activates the acupuncture meridians. As well as providing balance, it can strengthen internal organs, enhance power, reduce stress and promote relaxation and healing. Helps in injury prevention and can help injured parts to heal more quickly.

<u>Raspberry Leaf</u> – As well as women's health; Raspberry leaf tea is known to benefit the male reproductive system by detoxifying excess estrogen and balancing hormones. This can lead to better fertility and overall health as it promotes testosterone in men.

Raspberry leaf tea contains potassium which is excellent in reducing blood pressure. Lower blood pressure also can protect the cardiovascular system against serious heart complaints.

Raspberry leaf tea is an anti-inflammatory agent. Symptoms such as headaches, arthritis, fever, gastrointestinal issues may be caused by Inflammation. Raspberry leaf tea effectively soothes these symptoms.

Raspberry leaf tea supports a faster metabolism, which can aid weight loss. It can not only give you more energy but also help you to feel full while delivering vitamins, minerals, and key anti-oxidants.

Raspberry leaf tea contains tannins which give it an astringent property when used topically. Sunburns, eczema, rashes all benefit from an infusion of raspberry tea applied externally. For cold sores or gum disease, use as a mouthwash to reduce symptoms.

All of the health benefits listed above improve overall health and well-being; this impacts the body and mind in positive ways.

<u>Red clover</u> belongs to the legume family just like burdock root; it has similar characteristics to support healthy skin. It works gently to encourage detoxification in a number of ways: improved blood circulation, liver stimulation, and lymphatic cleansing. Red clover is also rich in nutrients and may improve hormone health. Use the blossoms in tea and other preparations. It is originally native to central Asia, Europe, and is now spread across many regions of the world.

In a similar way, to other legumes, red clover can fix nitrogen in the soil and help to repair damaged soils, which is why farmers love it. It has also been used for centuries as medicine, especially for skin conditions and the bronchial system.

- Another traditional use of red clover is for respiratory issues. Its antispasmodic properties and action as a mild sedative is the reason why it has been used for everything from coughs and bronchitis to asthma.

- While the leaf of the plant can be used in herbal medicine, the flowering top is the most beneficial and most used part. It contains many easily assimilated nutrients including calcium, beta-carotene, magnesium, manganese, zinc, copper, selenium, phosphorus, and potassium. Red clover also contains vitamin C and several B vitamins. Red clover can be used to make a tea by itself or with other nutritive herbs to help with nutrient deficiencies. Along with all its nutrients, red clover contains compounds called isoflavones.

- Isoflavones are a type of phytoestrogen, which can act similarly to estrogen in the body. How exactly isoflavones work in the body is still unknown, but they can be beneficial for hormone imbalances. One theory is that isoflavones bind to estrogen receptor sites and prevent estradiol and excess estrogen from accumulating. This effect is one of the reasons red clover features in herbal blends to balance hormones and enhance fertility.

- One of the most traditional uses for red clover is to help relieve menopausal symptoms. The phytoestrogens (isoflavones) in red clover are the main reason for this, helping to bring hormones back in balance. It is used to help with hot flashes, mood swings, and night sweats in particular. Red clover also has the potential to help reduce the loss of bone density because of its phytoestrogen content. One study using a red clover derived supplement found that women taking the supplement had significantly less bone density loss than the placebo group.

- Another common use of red clover is to support healthy skin and to help with conditions like eczema, psoriasis, and skin irritations. It can be used to make a skin wash that is used externally to soothe skin. But many of red clover's benefits for skin come from its cleansing effects on the blood and lymphatic system. These purifying properties assist the body, blood to get rid of wastes and toxins that may be responsible for the skin conditions.

A tea made with red clover (sometimes combined with nettle leaf or raspberry leaf) can be taken regularly to support the functions mentioned. It can be taken as a herbal tea to detoxify the body or as an extract to detoxify, assist with a cleanse of toxins out of the body that may be causing skin issues.

The list of healing benefits of red clover goes on.

Red clover's hormone balancing properties make it beneficial for relieving problematic menstrual symptoms and also for enhancing libido.

Research also shows that the isoflavones in red clover may help to prevent certain diseases to their anti carcinogenic abilities. It can also be used to clear lymphatic congestion and can provide overall immune support because of its many nutrients and active compounds. While red clover is available as a supplement and extract, it's most often used in herbal medicine as a tea.

Red clover is a very safe herb to use, even for a long period of time.

However, the phytoestrogens in red clover mean that it should be avoided by those with hormone or estrogen-sensitive disorders or any other hormone-sensitive conditions.

Red clover also has blood-thinning properties and should not be taken with other blood thinners and some heart medications.

<u>Reflexology</u> is a type of massage that involves applying different amounts of pressure to the feet, hands, and ears. It's based on a theory that these body parts are connected to certain organs and body systems. The practitioners of this technique are called reflexologists. Reflexology works to unblock certain channels in the body to provide a release for trauma and so promotes healing.

<u>Reiki</u> is a Japanese technique used for stress reduction and relaxation that also promotes healing. It is administered by "laying on hands" on the blocked body areas and is based on the idea that an unseen "life force energy" flows through the body and is the energy responsible for life. Reiki is very beneficial in healing a person from traumas and various different ailments if you are open to its benefits.

<u>Rosemary</u> is an evergreen shrub, popularly used herb in cooking. The medicinal uses of Rosemary have been praised for centuries, all over the world but scientific research has only recently corroborated these claims. Initial research affirms rosemary as an important addition to the diet, as it contains a wide variety of nutrients that are essential for health, such folate, manganese, pantothenic acid, niacin, thiamin and riboflavin. Rosemary is particularly rich in phytochemicals. Although phytochemicals are not as essential for survival as vitamins and minerals are, they are nevertheless important for fighting disease and maintaining overall health.

Health benefits of Rosemary are as follows:

- Its anti-oxidants and anti-inflammatory compounds;
- Ability to enhance memory and concentration;

- Its compounds prevent brain aging;

- It improves immune function;

- It protects against macular degeneration;

- Improving digestion abilities;

- Enhanced neurological protection;

- The hair oil is used to help hair grow;

<u>Saffron</u> – This plant is rich in anti-oxidants, the flavonoids in saffron protect against fungal infections. Due to its ability to produce serotonin; this chemical acts as a mood stabiliser, improves depression; curbs the appetite, reduces food cravings, aids weight loss and provides relief for pms symptoms.

<u>Sea Kelp</u> – If you are deficient in iodine this seaweed is beneficial in restoring iodine levels especially when taken with selenium rich foods. Sea Kelp also binds heavy metals and is rich in nutrients.

<u>Selenium deficiency</u> can cause problems with teeth, muscles, and hormones. Some soils are now lacking this important mineral. A large part of the thyroid gland requires this mineral; selenium is important as it aids in the utilisation of iodine, so it very beneficial for all thyroid functions.

<u>Sensitive teeth</u> can be remineralised by gently massaging teeth and gums with mustard oil; with its anti-bacterial and anti-inflammatory properties and Himalayan salt, at least twice a day. A noticeable difference can be noticed within a week. Moringa has beneficial properties such collagen renewal and anti-bacterial qualities so it may improve teeth and gum health when rubbed gently into the gums regularly. MSM is useful in restoring gum health.

Two acupressure points may help sensitivity in teeth, these are small intestine 18, located in the groove of the teeth to release energy blockages.

<u>Shatavari</u> – This is a hormonal balancing ayurvedic herb especially used as an aid for women's health. Shatavari is used as a good reproductive tonic. It is a go-to herb for concerns about loss of

libido, impotence, inflammation in sexual organs, and other sex-related concerns. It is highly effective as well for male reproductive health. Some of its attributes include its unctuous properties that cause an increase in reproductive fluids. Shatavari assists in the relief of pain from rheumatism and muscle spasms. It may be used as an aid to balance acid digestion and enhance alertness as well as fight stress.

Serotonin (also known as 5-hydroxytryptamine or 5-HT) is a naturally occurring substance; the main function of serotonin is as a neurotransmitter and to carry signals between nerve cells (called neurons) throughout your body.

Most commonly, serotonin is known for its role in the central nervous system (CNS). In the brain, serotonin helps with mood regulation and memory, but this essential neurotransmitter also has important jobs in other parts of the body.

In fact, most of the serotonin in your body can be found in your gut, not your brain. The intestines produce almost all of the body's serotonin supply; serotonin is required there to promote healthy digestion. Elsewhere in the body; serotonin assists with problems related to sleep, sexual function, bone health, and blood clotting. Due to its effect on mood it is often used in medicine to treat anxiety, depression and other mood disorders. Serotonin plays an important function in sleep as it converts to melatonin. A decrease in this neurotransmitter can affect sleep patterns.

Shea butter – Mainly due to its high concentration of vitamins and fatty acids, shea butter has been used as a cosmetic ingredient for centuries. It is technically a tree nut product, although, it is very low in the proteins that can trigger allergies and hasn't been known to cause allergies.

Shea butter is mainly used for its moisturising effects. These benefits are typically due to the butter's fatty acid content, holding the moisture in and reducing risk of dryness to skin. The butter is fully absorbed and no oily residue is left behind on the skin. This is due to shea butter's concentration of linoleic acid and oleic acid. The plant esters of this butter have been found to have anti-inflammatory properties. When used on the skin, it reduces Irritation caused by environmental factors; dry weather; as well as inflammatory skin conditions, such as eczema.

Shea is known for its strong anti-oxidant activity due to its content of significant levels of vitamins A and E. Anti-oxidants are important anti-ageing agents and they protect skin cells from free radicals that lead to premature ageing and dull-looking skin. It's also anti-bacterial, because of this topical application it may decrease the amount of acne causing bacteria on the skin, as it is also anti-fungal.

Shea tree products are powerful ingredients used to fight skin infections caused by fungi in some countries. As shea is known to kill spores of the fungi that causes ringworm and athlete's foot. It may prevent acne as shea butter is rich in different kinds of fatty acids. This composition helps clear the skin of excess oil (sebum). It can restore moisture to skin and lock it in to the epidermis, so skin doesn't dry out or feel "stripped" of oil. This results in a restoration of the natural balance of oils in the skin, which may put a stop to acne before it starts. It can help boost collagen production. Naturally occurring chemical compounds in the butter are thought to deactivate collagen fibre destruction and may minimise the appearance of fine lines and result in plumper skin. Both of its moisturising and anti-oxidant properties assist the skin in the regeneration of healthy new skin cells. With the right moisture balance on the surface of the skin, there are fewer dead skin cells in the way of fresh cell regeneration in the epidermis. Shea butter may reduce the appearance of stretch marks and scarring, as some use of shea butter stops scar tissue from reproducing, while encouraging healthy cell growth to take their place. This may help the skin heal and minimise the appearance of stretch marks and scarring. It may reduce photo ageing; the wrinkles and fine lines that environmental stress and ageing can create on skin.

Shirodhara is an ancient ayurvedic treatment conceived to ease physiological stress and mental fatigue. This treatment assists one to find harmony within the mind, body and spirit for holistic wellbeing and it is one of the most essential therapies mentioned in Ayurveda after meditation. This process of treatment can also rejuvenate and purify the body and treat several disorders. It balances the individual constitutions in the body and enhances the functioning of the nervous system.

This process involves pouring a steady stream of warm oil onto the forehead for a half an hour to promote calmness and general well-being. This therapy is an ideal treatment for reducing high levels of mental stress as it induces calmness, promotes tranquility, and facilitates relaxation. The steady pour of warm oil brings about a relaxation response where the body enters deep relaxation, stress hormones decline while hyper-alert brain patterns (beta waves) transition into more relaxed-alert ones (alpha waves). The relaxation response is the body's way of turning on the parasympathetic nervous system, that part of the nervous system which conserves energy, slows heart rate, and relaxes muscles. A small study showed the shirodhara treatment significantly affects those measurable markers of relaxation by decreasing respiration rate, reducing diastolic blood pressure, and slowing heart rate.

Given that most modern disease has some link to stress, minimising its impact is valuable for generating lifelong heath. The relaxation response directly counteracts stress by reversing its physical effects. Each session of shirodhara treatment may invoke such a powerful relaxation response that the effects of stress are mitigated for days. Although, there may be some tiredness and processing after the sessions.

This form of Ayurvedic therapy is one of the steps involved in Panchakarma; a cleansing and detoxification process practiced to enable healing. The main objective of this treatment is to bring back balance. The Shirodhara treatment is recommended to relieve stress, anxiety, fatigue, migraine, depression, and improve vision. The common factor in all these conditions is the brain. Shirodhara works directly on the various nerves in the head that stimulate the areas of the brain, as the therapy offers a great sense of relaxation and induces soothing effects on the mind and body. It uses several Ayurvedic oils that not only soothe and nourish the brain, but also treat a host of health anomalies, like anxiety, depression, fatigue, insomnia, stress, migraine, hypertension, and more.

Shirodhara treatment has been shown to reduce brain waves to the more relaxed alpha state, similar to the effects of meditation. So it stands to reason that this treatment has a beneficial impact on sleep quality. A small recent study found this treatment to be a successful option "to improve sleep quality and quality of life in persons with sleep problems." Not only is sleep quality improved with the shirodhara treatment, better health is also experienced. Shirodhara aims to calm and relax an overactive mind.

Sinus – An ayurvedic cleanse may assist chronic sinus problems; the cleanse involves pouring a saline solution through each nostril until the solution pours out of the opposite nostril. Nasya, (an ayurvedic treatment), with medicated oils or ghee or coconut oil can prove very beneficial for sinus, it helps the nervous system, it protects against allergens such as pollen as it lubricates the nasal passages.

Sinus issues can be linked to the elocaecial valve and the intestines. Gentle massage may assist here. Anulom Vilom and bramri pranayama can reduce the symptoms. Acupressure points are located on fingertips when gentle pressure is applied to fingers and thumb; obstructions in the body are removed and the blocked sinuses are N-acetylcysteine can also play a vital role in boosting the body's immune system, as it has been used to help dissolve mucus in those suffering from chronic respiratory complaints. Probiotics are also useful to restore healthy gut bacteria, which can eliminate unhealthy microbes.

Skin – Massage skin in the morning with almond oil, before taking a shower and keep skin clean and hydrated. Regular cold showers offer many health benefits including improved skin conditions. Eat lots of fresh fruit and vegetables every day and drink plenty of good quality water. Ensure consumption of good healthy fats to keep skin and muscles toned and healthy.

Sore throat – A salt water gargle a few times a day and a gentle neck massage with almond oil will relieve a sore throat and other associated symptoms of coughs and colds.

Spirulina is a blue-green algae and Spirulina is very rich in chlorophyll, just like chlorella. It's one of the most nutrient dense foods around that binds to toxins when consumed, carrying them out of the body. Spirulina also contains a powerful anti-oxidant known as phycocyanin that supports liver and kidney function, further promoting detoxification. It is used regularly to assist as a body cleanse.

<u>Stomach ulcer</u> – Remedies include aniseed, bhringraj and triphala. A drink of water combined with salt will ease acidity.

<u>Stress</u> – The stress reduction benefits of Shirodhara have been discussed in depth. Over time the stress reducing, calming and curative effects of Shirodhara are felt; seek advice from an ayurvedic qualified therapist. Walks in nature and generally being around nature induce a release from stress. Breathing properly and taking time out can also have very positive effects on stress management. Different relaxation modalities such as ayurvedic treatments, yoga, meditation and mindfulness and Epsom salt baths all induce a sense of relaxation to the mind and body thereby decreasing high stress levels. Quiet assists stress reduction as noise contributes to increasing stress levels.

<u>Stretch marks</u> – Gotu Kola, should only be used fortnightly with a fortnight break, as prolonged use may cause side effects. With regular use loose and saggy skin is improved.

It boosts the formation of collagen and skin tissue and is crucial in maintaining skin elasticity and youthful skin. Castor oil is also beneficial in collagen production. The stretch marks on skin can be repaired by regular application of Shea butter due to its beneficial nutrients.

<u>Sugar Cravings</u> – This may indicate a chromium deficiency. Blackstrap molasses are a rich source of chromium. Sugar cravings also can be reduced by eating a balanced meal including carbohydrates, protein etc, on a timely basis and by not skipping meals.

<u>Sunburn</u> – Apply a paste of water and triphala. Alternatively apply fresh aloe vera gel.

<u>Sunflower seeds</u> – These seeds are great at reducing inflammation; are rich in vitamins and minerals and have a high oil content.

<u>Sunlight</u> is very important, so try and get out in the sun if you can avoid getting sun burnt. It is a good source of vitamin D and assists general well-being and mood.

<u>Suntan removal</u> – Apply sugar, honey and lemon juice.

<u>Tai Chi</u>, is sometimes also known as "Shadowboxing". Tai chi is an internal Chinese martial art practiced for defence training, health

benefits, and as an aid to meditation. Tai chi is a system of movements and positions believed to have developed in 12th Century China. Tai chi techniques aim to address the body and mind as an integral system and are traditionally believed to have mental and physical health benefits. Various research suggests tai chi offers a range of benefits for people with and without chronic conditions. These benefits include:

- improved balance

- pain management

- improved brain function

- and improved sleep quality

<u>Teeth</u> – Oil pulling with Coconut oil will naturally whiten teeth, maintain good oral health and healthy teeth. Salt may be included with the oil to strengthen the enamel and reduce inflammation. Remineralise teeth by rubbing salt/moringa/spirulina (sea weed)/ triphala into the teeth and gums daily. With the many health benefits of cloves. Clove oil/cloves are useful with the relief of the pain of toothache due its antiseptic and anti-bacterial qualities. Clove oil has been used for thousands of years with records from the ancient Roman civilizations using it to relieve dental pain and freshen up their breath, treat gum disease and sores. It has also been used in Ayurvedic medicine for centuries for the same purpose.

<u>Tension</u> – is normally released during regular exercise. Ujjayi pranayama is also known to reduce tension as it is very calming and it may reduce anxiety, do not attempt this if you have problems with your lungs.

<u>Thyme</u> The use of Thyme extends back to ancient Egyptian and Roman times. Thyme has remained popular over the years because of its health benefits, which are all owed to its diverse profile of vitamins, minerals, and other essential nutritional compounds. Thyme is an excellent source of fiber, calcium, iron, manganese, and vitamins A, B6, and C. There are also robust phenols inside the plant — thymol, eugenol, and carvacrol.

The health benefits of Thyme include its use as a bug repellant. It is resistant to harmful organisms. Thyme has powerful anti-oxidant abilities mainly due to the compounds it contains- thymol and carvacrol. Respiratory health is important, especially for those with compromised immune systems. Thyme supports normal respiratory health in every season. Research shows that thyme assists to soothe-the airways, coughs and colds and promote normal lung health.

Thyme contains nutrients that support normal blood pressure and cholesterol levels. Blood pressure and cholesterol both play a significant role in heart health.

Daily consumption of the herbs - thyme and oregano can influence neurotransmitters and boost your mood. One compound found in thyme oil, carvacrol, when consumed over a seven-day period, positively affected dopamine and serotonin status so a good mood booster and useful to maintain mental wellness.

Thyroid Health — Iron deficiency can impair the production of TSH (thyroid stimulating hormone) and contribute to hypothyroidism.

The thyroid requires iodine, selenium and also iron to function properly and other trace minerals. TSH, is a hormone produced by the pituitary gland. The pituitary is always in communication with the thyroid. Without proper TSH production, the thyroid gland receives none of the signs that are necessary for the production of T3 (triiodothyronine) and T4 (thyroxine). In fact, reports indicate that patients undergoing thyroid hormone replacement therapy get better results when they're also given iron (as opposed to thyroid hormone therapy by itself). A good natural source of iron is nettle leaf, which is a rich source of iron, as it has traditionally been used in the treatment of anemia. So, including nettles in the diet could be a good way to naturally boost iron and support the thyroid.

Tiger milk mushroom — This mushroom has been used for hundreds of years as a health tonic by the aborigines for its healing properties on many medical ailments as well as a general tonic to strengthen the body. Scientists have successfully cultivated and studied Tiger Mushroom to confirm its safety and medicinal properties. It is known for its traditional use to support lung and respiratory health and allergy reduction, as well as to boost immunity in general.

Tongue scraping — This reduces the build-up on the tongue. This practice daily assists in the removal of bacteria, fungus, toxins, dead cells and food. It assists in the prevention of prevent bad breath, gum disease, cavities etc. Scraping the tongue each morning prevents re-absorption of toxins the body has been trying to expel. It is important to get rid of these toxins otherwise if may lead to ill health. Tongue scraping it is said can give the internal organs a gentle massage, as it is suggested various internal organs are linked to the tongue. The back of the tongue corresponds with the colon, it aids in the movement of food through the intestine. Use a stainless-steel tongue scraper, as stainless steel is anti-bacterial.

<u>TCM</u> – Traditional Chinese medicine is thousands of years old. It is based on the principle that a vital force of life Qi surges through the body. An imbalance to Qi can cause serious disease and illness. This imbalance is thought to be caused by a dissension in the opposite and complementary forces that make up the Qi. These are called yin and yang. The ancient chinese believed that humans are microcosms of the larger surrounding universe or macrocosm, and are interconnected with nature and subject to its forces. Balance between health and disease is a key concept. TCM treatment seeks to restore this balance through treatment specific to the individual as it is believed that to regain balance; you must achieve the balance between the internal body organs and the external elements of earth, fire, water, wood, and metal. Treatment to regain balance may involve:

- Acupuncture
- Cupping (warmed glass jars used to create suction on certain points of the body)
- Herbal remedies
- Massage
- Movement and concentration exercises (tai chi)
- Moxibustion (herbal leaves burning on or near the body)

<u>Triphala</u> is an ayurvedic blend of three important herbs. Some of its benefits include the ability to boost immunity, fight infections, rejuvenate the body and strengthen organs. It protects against tooth decay as it reduces the production of plaque. Triphala protects against dental problems, as the build-up of dental plaque is a precursor to cavities, gum disease, and other dental health issues. Triphala can help you avoid these issues all thanks to its antimicrobial properties. One study found that it was, in fact,

able to protect the gums from free radical damage better than commercial toothpastes. Triphala also helps manage gastric ulcers, diabetes, and urinary tract infections. In ancient times, an eye bath using triphala was used to help eye ailments due to its anti-fungal and antimicrobial effects. It can be used to heal the stomach and also to get rid of anything unhealthy and toxic in the digestive tract. Triphala also helps to boost Immunity and fights infections. Ancient ayurvedic practitioners suggest having triphala along with honey and ghee (aid absorption) – a treatment known as triphala rasayana – every day for longevity and good health. Studies have revealed the combination of herbs that make up triphala are effective against a range of pathogens; which include common causes of infection like E. coli, some types of Salmonella, and various types of Staphylococcus bacteria, to name a few. Taking triphala every day may help ward off such infections and keep you healthy.

<u>Tulsi</u> – This herb is known as a satvic plant (health giving), in ayurvedic medicine. Ancient eastern scriptures refer to Tulsi as the most sacred plant in the world. A positive herb it is difficult to find all the qualities and benefits of Tulsi in any other plants. It aims to support healthy immune, blood, lymphatic and respiratory systems, as well as reduce congestion, support the lungs and assist healthy breathing. It is a calming and stress reducing plant and can even reverse the effects of stress and aid the body's ability to regenerate. It is able to penetrate deep into all the bodily tissues and pull out the environmental stressors such as pollution, heavy metals and other toxins. Tulsi removes toxic heavy metals and other toxins from the blood brain barrier in a similar way to dulse and MSM.

<u>Turmeric</u> – It should be taken as a whole herb, not various extracts such as curcumin as strong doses of this extract may cause health issues. Turmeric is a very beneficial herb as it reduces inflammation in the body and offers many healing properties. It is known to reduce cholesterol and arthritis pain. Turmeric improves brain functions and supports cognitive performance as it has enhanced neuro-protective properties. It supports cardiovascular health, age related degenerative conditions. Turmeric protects the DNA from permanent damage.

<u>Ujjayi Breathing</u> – This practice is calming and stress reducing; throughout the inhalation and exhalation breaths ventilation is managed during the rest in breathing, it is at the point the real work of tuning the nervous system occurs. Nasal laterality during this practice serves to further challenge co-ordination of breathing and the brain. It also serves to stimulate each hemisphere of the brain independently as well as alternating stimulus of the sympathetic (inhalation) and parasympathetic (exhalation) nervous systems in a similar manner to the effects of light meditation. It can be beneficial for the sinuses, thyroid gland, respiratory system, amongst other functions as it strengthens the lungs and boosts vitality. Ujjayi breath works to balance the energy channels to promote healing and harmonise the endocrine system.

The parasympathetic nervous system (PSNS), is part of the nervous system that sends signals to and from different body parts via nerves and is responsible for all the bodily activities that take place during rest. Due to the deliberate constriction of the glottis during this practice and its influence on the vagus nerve it serves a variety of PSNS functions such as to innervate the heart, lungs, esophagus, stomach, liver, kidneys and pancreas. The stimulus of this system tends to lower heart rate and respiration.

The counterpart of the PSNS is the sympathetic nervous system (SNS), which is responsible for "fear, fight or flight" activities that occur when in danger or during overstressed situations. Ujjayi assists to alleviate these symptoms, manage over activity as the mind is calmed during this pranayama practice bringing about a more restful relaxed state. As with all pranayama practices caution is advised and these practices should be learnt from a suitably qualified practitioner.

<u>Vicarious Trauma</u> – A form of trauma related to taking on indirect trauma from dealing directly with victim's trauma.

<u>Vitamins and minerals</u> are sometimes referred to as anti-oxidants and are nutrients your body needs in small amounts to work properly and stay healthy. Most of the nutrients can be found in a varied and balanced diet, although some people may need to take extra supplements. For example <u>Vitamin D</u>– It is of vital importance to health as it is an essential nutrient. Vitamin D helps regulate the amount of calcium and phosphate in the body. These nutrients are

needed to keep bones, teeth and muscles healthy. A lack of vitamin D can lead to bone deformities such as rickets in children, and bone related conditions in adults. Natural sources of Vitamin D are sunlight, mushrooms, fortified milks and tofu.

<u>Walnuts</u> – The nuts and the husk are soaked in water for a few hours until the water becomes a very dark colour; after removing the nuts, this water may be applied to hair as a final rinse to colour grey hairs. Benefits of consuming walnuts include, maintenance of brain health, and protection of arteries as walnuts are a rich source of omega 3 fatty acids. Due to the anti-inflammatory properties of omega 3 acids regular consumption of these nuts builds immunity. They are also an effective cure for insomnia and gut health.

<u>Water</u> – Drink enough good quality water throughout the day to flush out toxins and assist digestion. It is important to stay hydrated for all bodily functions. Health problems can occur due to dehydration.

<u>Weight loss</u> – Eat a healthy diet avoid refined sugar and fried foods. Eat more fresh fruit and vegetables and healthy fats. Eat meals on time, avoid snacking in between meals, and also eat a healthy portion size this will help with gradual weight loss use a plate as a guide. Do not miss meals as hormones become imbalanced and cravings for junk food can occur. Daily exercise even brisk walking approximately twenty minutes per day. This activity may be used to support and become part of a weight loss program. Being active is essential to weight loss. Take up a new activity; ensure a good night's sleep to help with moods.

<u>Women's health</u> – Shatavari is considered a supreme tonic and hormonal balancer for women's health. It is known to support women through every stage of life. Shatavari's main constituents are steroidal saponins, hence its use as an estrogen regulator. This modulation helps to regulate menstrual cycles, manage PMS symptoms, alleviate menstrual cramps and control the amount of blood lost. Shatavari greatly helps with fluid retention and may be helpful with the uncomfortable bloating before a period. This versatile herb is useful for women with fertility issues as it lines and protects the cervix. It can protect against miscarriage. Due to its oily, heavy nature, Shatavari nourishes the female reproductive system from within to relieve menopausal symptoms such as vaginal dryness, hot flashes and

insomnia. This phytoestrogen-rich herb naturally helps to balance the hormones responsible for many of the more unpleasant symptoms during this change in life. Shatavari also stimulates and balances the mood enhancing hormones; endorphins, serotonin and dopamine - so it can greatly reduce mood swings, irritability and menopause induced depression. It may also act as an aphrodisiac.

Maca is also useful in balancing hormones and often assists with the regulation of irregular periods as well menopausal symptoms. MSM specially has several benefits. It helps in balancing hormones and controlling the activity of enzymes in the body.

<u>Wounds</u> – Zinc is beneficial for healing damaged tissue and wounds. Aloe vera gel applied to burns and wounds is very soothing and healing.

<u>Wrinkles</u> – Apply a mix of shatavari root to reduce/clear wrinkles. Shatavari root can be used with Castor/Sesame oil to maintain hydration and youthful skin.

<u>Xerosis</u> – This condition causes abnormal dryness of skin/mucous membranes. It may be remedied by using coconut oil or shea butter as these products replenish some of the lost oils from bathing. Castor oil and ghee can also be used.

<u>Yarrow</u> is considered a medicinal herb. Yarrow is commonly used for wounds, skin, liver disorders, diarrhea, gas, colds, asthma, runny nose, arthritis and has many more uses.

<u>Yoga</u> improves mental health. Over time yoga builds full body strength, balance, flexibility as well as resilience. Yoga decreases inflammation in the body and brings a sense of relief to back pain and arthritis pain. It can support heart health, assist relaxation, reduce anxiety, reduce depression and decrease and improve sleep problems. Yoga, meditation and mindfulness practices together all assist in stress management. Breathing slow full deep relaxing breaths and long deep exhalations release stress.

<u>Zinc</u> – This important trace mineral is essential to most functions in the body; it is necessary for almost 100 enzymes to carry out vital chemical reactions. Zinc is used to aid fertility, improve digestion and it is beneficial for healing wounds. Zinc plays a major part in

the creation of DNA, growth of cells, building of proteins, healing damaged tissue and supporting a healthy immune system. Due to this zinc supports a decrease in the incidence of pneumonia with its good immune booster potential as the duration of colds and flu are also reduced by a day. It is used to assist eye-care, hair health and zinc has many other beneficial attributes. Green beans, peas, potatoes, seeds and whole-grains are all good natural food sources of zinc.

Only take supplements on the advice of health professionals, they can check on any potential side effects or interactions with medications, foods, or other herbs and supplements. They can advise you on the suitability of the supplement or any associated risks. Do not take any chances with supplements if you are pregnant or breastfeeding.

www.ingramcontent.com/pod-product-compliance
Lightning Source LLC
Chambersburg PA
CBHW031407250726
48656CB00002B/568